FOREWORD

This is the second of the Government's reports on heavy metals to be published in the Pollution Paper series. It concerns mercury.

Many of us are aware of the environmental impact of mercury in the context of what has become known as 'Minamata Disease'. This type of disaster, which occurred in Japan – and which led to deaths and disablement – has not been seen elsewhere. But it is nonetheless important for us to be aware of our own situation with respect to pollution of the environment by mercury. This is the purpose of this report.

The report is reassuring in that it shows that most of us are only exposed to mercury levels well below what is considered acceptable by international experts. In recent years the use of mercury in certain applications has become more rigorously controlled, or has been deliberately reduced; and the disposal of mercury-containing wastes has likewise been subjected to greater control. Monitoring programmes have also been extended and co-ordinated.

The Government accept the view expressed in this report that, whilst there is no evidence to cause concern for public health, it would be prudent to keep man's total intake of mercury as low as practicable. This means that, although there is no need for urgent action, the opportunity to reduce exposure should be taken as and when appropriate, taking account of industrial economic viability, the technical adequacy of alternative technologies and the availability of less hazardous substitutes.

The effects of undue exposure to mercury can be serious. The essentially precautionary approach set out above is thus amply justified. And it should ensure our protection from this particular environmental hazard.

PETER SHORE
Secretary of State for the Environment

CONTENTS

DEPARTMENT OF THE ENVIRONMENT

CENTRAL UNIT ON ENVIRONMENTAL POLLUTION

ENVIRONMENTAL MERCURY AND MAN

*A Report of an Inter-Departmental
Working Group on Heavy Metals*

Pollution Paper No. 10

LONDON

HER MAJESTY'S STATIONERY OFFICE

This is one of a series of papers to be published for the Department of the Environment on various aspects of pollution. The previous reports were:

1. The Monitoring of the Environment in the United Kingdom (HMSO, 1974)
2. Lead in the Environment and its Significance to Man (HMSO, 1974)
3. The Non-Agricultural Uses of Pesticides in Great Britain (HMSO, 1974)
4. Controlling Pollution (HMSO, 1975)
5. Chlorofluorocarbons and their Effect on Stratospheric Ozone (HMSO, 1976)
6. The Separation of Oil from Water for North Sea Oil Operations (HMSO, 1976)
7. Effects of Airborne Sulphur Compounds on Forests and Freshwaters (HMSO, 1976)
8. Accidental Oil Pollution of the Sea (HMSO, 1976)
9. Pollution Control in Great Britain: How it Works (HMSO, 1976)

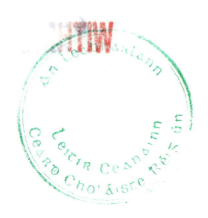

v

SUMMARY

I. Mercury is present in trace quantities in all parts of the environment. This is a consequence of emissions from both natural sources of mercury and from man's industrial use of mercury and its compounds. The major natural sources are volcanic action and weathering of Earth's crustal materials, which together possibly release each year up to about 150,000 tonnes of mercury to air and to rain, freshwaters and the seas and thence to soils, sediments, plants and animals.

II. Mercury is used in the chemicals industry, in production of chlorine and alkalis and in catalysis and paints, in agriculture and related areas, and in pharmaceuticals, dentistry and the electrical industry. About 9,000 tonnes annually have been used world-wide and over the last decade the UK has used between 235 and 788 tonnes each year. Each of these uses may give rise to emissions to the general environment; emissions may also arise from, for example, the burning of fossil fuels, metal processing and disposal of mercury-containing wastes. The total quantity of mercury mobilised by man's activities is much smaller than that mobilised naturally, but emissions as a result of man's activities may nevertheless be important because they may result in high local concentrations of mercury.

III. Food is the major source of exposure to mercury for most people, i.e. those not occupationally exposed. In the UK, the average dietary intake totals 5–10 microgrammes daily (0·035–0·070 milligrammes weekly) of which 2–5 micro-grammes daily (0·014–0·035 milligrammes weekly) may be in the form of methylmercury compounds. It is reassuring that this level of intake is well within the provisional tolerable intake of 0·30 milligrammes (total mercury) per person per week (of which not more than 0·20 milligrammes should be in the methyl form) proposed by the Food and Agriculture Organisation and the World Health Organisation. Furthermore, there is no evidence that our dietary intake of mercury is increasing. Of the various foods we eat, fish is important in relation to mercury intake; this is because natural processes occurring in sediments can convert all forms of mercury, including those derived from industrial discharges, into methylmercury compounds, which are readily transported and accumulated through the aquatic food chain to edible fish. (The reverse reaction, converting these compounds into methane and volatile inorganic mercury compounds also occurs.) Ingested methylmercury compounds are almost completely absorbed in man, but excreted only very slowly; they can, if taken in large enough quantities cause irreversible damage to the central nervous system. Because of these qualities, methylmercury compounds are potentially the most hazardous form of mercury.

IV. Children are not especially at risk of developing mercury poisoning. However, it has been thought prudent to control the mercury content of paints for use on pens, pencils and brushes, since these might be chewed by children. Such paints are subject to a maximum soluble mercury content of 100 parts per million (as are the cores of such instruments) under the Pencils and Graphic Instruments (Safety) Regulations 1974; the Toys (Safety) Regulations 1974 prescribe the same limits for paints to be used on toys.

V. There are no regulations made under the Factories Act to require the medical examination of those working with mercury. Nevertheless, many workers are screened by the Employment Medical Advisory Service by clinical assessment and analysis of urine. Poisoning by mercury as a consequence of employment, when it occurs in a place of employment to which the Factories Act 1961 applies, has to be notified to the Chief Inspector of Factories. In its clinically apparent stage it is a rare condition, the total number of cases in the UK varying from 0 to 6 annually over the last half century. However, urine analysis shows that there are many cases of high mercury absorption that are not notified, because the clinical symptoms are not sufficiently developed to warrant them being defined as mercury poisoning. The health of people working in dental practices, where exposure to mercury could be higher than average, is now the responsibility of the Health and Safety Commission. The British Dental Association has provided its members with advice on control of exposure to mercury.

VI. The use of mercury in certain applications has been deliberately reduced in recent years. In the paper and pulp industry, the use of mercurial slimicides in the UK was eliminated several years ago and the use of mercurial fungicides in adhesives is now very small. Agricultural and related uses, which now account for about 5 per cent of total identified mercury usage in the UK, have also declined, and what is used is generally in the form of less toxic compounds. The production of chlorine and alkalis, which uses more mercury than any other activity, has been responsible for the greatest emissions of metallic and inorganic mercury, but the industry has taken and is taking steps to reduce emissions by installation of treatment processes, as far as is practicable. The major producer has indicated to Government that it plans to use the alternative diaphragm process, which uses no mercury, in future production plant in the United Kingdom.

VII. The Control of Pollution Act 1974, when fully implemented, will extend the powers of regional water authorities to control the discharge of toxic materials, including mercury, to river and coastal waters; it has already empowered local authorities in England and Wales to control disposal of wastes on land by a system of licensing (in Scotland, control is still achieved through the Deposit of Poisonous Wastes Act). A special Working Group has been set up to consider especially hazardous materials, including those containing mercury, and it will report shortly, providing a Code of Practice on the disposal of these materials. The Dumping at Sea Act 1974 prohibits the dumping of any substance at sea except by licence. A licence is not granted for mercury and its compounds except where they are present as trace contaminants of e.g. sewage sludges and harbour dredgings. Under a recently agreed Directive, Member States of the EEC are required to eliminate pollution by mercury and its compounds in inland surface waters, territorial waters, coastal waters and ground waters.

VIII. Action is being taken by the Government to improve the monitoring of our environment. In accordance with recommendations made in the report "The Monitoring of the Environment in the United Kingdom" (HMSO, 1974a, Pollution Paper No. 1), Pollution Monitoring Management Groups have been established to consider monitoring needs in relation to air, freshwater, the marine environment and land; and biological and human health. Monitoring for mercury in air has been initiated by the Air Pollution Monitoring Management Group at sites likely to be contaminated by this metal and a harmonised water quality monitoring programme has been set up, now under the guidance of the Freshwater Monitoring Management Group, to sample all major rivers and tributaries; both initiatives are already providing data. The Marine Pollution Monitoring Management Group includes mercury as one of the substances to be measured in its monitoring programme. The surveillance of foodstuffs for heavy metals, including mercury, continues under the direction of the Steering Group on Food Surveillance through its Working Party on the Monitoring of Foodstuffs for Heavy Metals. The Government also sponsors research to improve our knowledge of the release and dispersal of mercury, the pathways by which it is transported from one part of the environment to another and its effects on plant and animal life, including man.

IX. The conclusions which have emerged for this appraisal are reassuring. The average exposure of people in the UK to the major source of mercury (food) is well within the provisional tolerable limit proposed by the Food and Agriculture Organisation and World Health Organisation, but special consideration should continue of those who might be more exposed, e.g. from unusual diets, or the air, and of those in whom medical disorders might produce a low tolerance to mercury. Mercury is a toxic substance having no known function in human biochemistry or physiology. It is desirable on health grounds that man's total intake of mercury be kept as low as practicable. Precipitate action is clearly not called for and would result in significant economic and social costs. On the other hand, where contamination by mercury exists or is likely to arise, action progressively to reduce man-made contributions should be taken as and when appropriate, taking account not only of the desirability of improving safety margins still further, but also of industrial economic viability, technical adequacy and the availability of less hazardous substitutes. Where a pathway is identified through which mercury can reach man, special care is needed; this may necessitate more stringent control over releases of mercury to the environment. Research is already in hand on development of less hazardous substitutes for some applications and liaison between industry and Government in a number of areas is already under way.

CHAPTER 1

ENVIRONMENTAL MERCURY

Introduction

1. This chapter outlines the reasons for current interest in the environmental significance of mercury, the relative magnitudes of sources of mercury arising both naturally and from man's activities, and the concentrations of mercury in various parts of the environment. A more detailed account appears in Appendix I.

2. The most important ore of mercury, its red sulphide 'cinnabar', has been known for thousands of years, being used as a pigment and as a therapeutic. Since medieval times, other compounds of mercury have been prepared and used in medicine for douching, irrigation of the bladder, in teething powders, laxatives or diuretics, and the metal itself was widely used in ointments for control of skin disorders and syphilis, but these uses have decreased substantially. Some of the symptoms associated with hazards to human health arising from the use of mercury, such as tremors, inflammation of the gums and general irritability have been recognised for a very long time and the term 'mercurialism' has been used to indicate intoxication (poisoning) by mercury or its compounds. Mercurialism has always been an occupational hazard amongst those mining the ore and amongst people working in mercury-using industries, but the incidence of poisoning today in the UK is very low. The Health and Safety Commission is responsible (through the Health and Safety Executive) for administration of legal requirements on occupational hazards and this topic is dealt with in more detail in Chapter 3.

3. Until the 1950s, no widespread hazard to animals or to people not occupationally exposed to mercury was known to exist. During the late 1950s, however, Swedish ornithologists (Borg et al, 1969) discovered that some species of birds, particularly raptors, were declining in numbers. This was attributed in part to consumption of cereal seeds treated with organic* mercury compounds by species which were then eaten by raptors. Cereal seed treatments with mercury compounds were devised in the late 1920s and were in widespread use in the UK by the mid-1930s. In the 1960s it was noticed that bird deaths sometimes occurred at the times when cereals were sown. These birds deaths, following

---

*In this report frequent reference is made to 'inorganic' and 'organic' forms of mercury. The term inorganic refers to compounds which do not contain (except in a very few cases) a mercury-carbon bond; inorganic compounds are thus, for our purposes, essentially relatively simple salts such as mercurous or mercuric chloride. Organic compounds do contain mercury-carbon bonds and there are three types of particular interest: these are the 'aryl' compounds, such as phenylmercury acetate, the 'alkyl' compounds such as dimethylmercury or ethylmercury chloride and the 'alkoxyalkyl' compounds such as ethoxymethylmercury chloride.

ingestion of treated seeds, have generally been attributed in the UK to organo-chlorine pesticides that were used in association with the mercury compounds, rather than to the mercury compounds themselves. High levels of mercury in fish in Sweden (and in birds feeding on them) were also attributed to the widespread use of mercury compounds as slimicides in pulp and paper mills.

4. Another hazard, of great immediate consequence to man, came to light in Japan and ultimately gave rise to the term 'Minamata Disease'. It arose from the massive and prolonged discharge of mercury compounds formed from catalysts used in acetaldehyde and vinyl chloride production to the waters of Minamata Bay. Here, natural processes probably converted some of the mercury content of effluents into methylmercury compounds, which are a particular hazard to health, although this form of mercury was also present in the discharge itself. The methylmercury compounds were then accumulated in the tissues of fish living and feeding in the bay. Since the diets of local fishermen and their families largely consisted of fish, many of these people had an excessively high intake of mercury, and in particular of methylmercury com-pounds. This incident resulted in the poisoning of 121 people, of whom 46 died, in the period 1953–1970 (Takeuchi, 1972a). Twenty-two infants with brain damage (palsy and retardation) were born to mothers who were mainly symptom-free and this indicates transplacental foetal damage and the possible concentration of methylmercury in the foetus (WHO, 1972). These unfortunate people, or their heirs, have recently been awarded financial compensation in the Japanese courts for injuries and disabilities resulting from exposure to mercury (Anon, 1973). By March 1975 there were 684 officially verified patients and 115 had died (Environment Agency, 1975). A similar incident occurred around the Agano River, Niigata, Japan, from 1965 onwards; in this case by March 1975 there were 516 certified victims of poisoning and 23 deaths (Environment Agency, 1975). A third outbreak of the disease has recently been reported (Japan Times, 1973) but this has not been confirmed (Environment Agency, 1975). In these incidents many domestic animals, particularly cats, were also affected as were fish, shellfish and seabirds. Disasters of this type or magnitude have not occurred in any other country, although recent reports (e.g. Smith and Smith, 1975) indicate the possible existence of a problem in Canada; having set a maximum limit on the concentration of mercury in fish, Sweden, Canada and the USA have thought it necessary to prohibit removal and sale of fish from certain of their waters on occasion.

5. Another source of severe damage to human health which occurred in Iraq, Pakistan, Guatemala and the USA arose from incidents involving the con-sumption of food containing high concentrations of mercury derived from alkylmercury agricultural seed-treatments. These treatments use organic com-pounds of mercury which are applied to seeds (e.g. grain etc.) to prevent seed-borne disease. In Iraq, treated seeds, intended for planting, had inadvertently been used to make bread (Bakir et al, 1973): in the USA, livestock was fed on treated grain, and then slaughtered for human consumption (Curley et al, 1971). In both instances, severe poisoning or death has occurred, particularly in Iraq,

2

where thousands were poisoned and hundreds died. Livestock was also affected. Several countries have now banned the use of alkylmercurial seed treatments and an international group of experts convened by the Food and Agriculture Organisation (FAO) and World Health Organisation (WHO) has recommended that their use should be restricted solely to treatment of nuclear stocks of cereal seed and never permitted for treatment of cereal seed to be exported for the production of food (WHO, 1974).

6. Very few incidents involving accidental feeding of dressed grain to livestock have occurred in the UK and in each case damage to human health was averted. In one case dressed seed was fed to hens and in another case to cows (Daykin, 1975). The particular usage of mercury responsible for the Minamata incident does not now exist in the UK, although of course industrial discharges containing mercury are made to water. The purpose of this report is to examine objectively the present situation in the UK with regard to exposure of the general public to mercury present in the environment and to evaluate its effect on human health. This has meant reviewing the use of mercury in the UK, the emissions of mercury from various industries and the available data on prevailing concentrations of mercury in most components of our environment. A summary of the findings and data for each area of use or particular part of the environment is given in the remaining paragraphs of this Chapter. Detailed information (together with references) is set out in Appendix I and Tables 1, 2 and 3.

7. It must be noted that drawing substantive conclusions from data on trace quantities of mercury in various parts of the environment is difficult and prone to uncertainty because of the technical problems which arise in chemical analysis for mercury and because of problems in comparing results from different techniques.

Natural mercury

8. Mercury occurs naturally in trace quantities in all components of the environment. A variety of natural processes are responsible for the transfer of mercury from one part of the environment to another: these include volcanic activity and degassing of crustal materials, both on land and under the sea; weathering of rocks etc. and sub-marine leaching; evaporation, rain and dustfall; and uptake of mercury from water, sediments and soils by plants and animals, followed by death, decay and leaching. Volcanic activity and degassing are by far the most important of these processes in terms of quantity of mercury mobilised, accounting for up to an estimated 150,000 tonnes* annually.

Industrial usage

9. In the UK, between 235 and 788 tonnes of mercury and mercury compounds have been used annually over the last decade. Such large variations arise principally because demand by the chloralkali industry, the major user, varies according to its needs for commissioning new plant. This industry produces

---

*1 tonne is 1 metric tonne = 1000 kilogrammes (kg), and is approximately equal to 1 Imperial ton.

chlorine, which is vital to the maintenance of wholesome water and for production of some plastics, and caustic soda, which is an important chemical used in many other industries. The principal uses of mercury (and the figures for 1975) are: the chloralkali industry – 475 tonnes supplied, 283 tonnes used; primary batteries – 80 tonnes; paints – 34 tonnes; agriculture and related uses – 28 tonnes; dentistry – 30 tonnes; electrical and control instruments – 14 tonnes; catalysis – 11 tonnes; laboratory chemicals – 10 tonnes; pharmaceuticals – 2 tonnes; adhesives – 1 tonne; and miscellaneous uses such as in munitions, pigments, photography, fireworks, laboratory vacuum pumps and textile fungicides, which taken together total about 6 tonnes.

Emissions

10. Each of the above uses can give rise to release of mercury to the environment. In addition, mercury occurs in trace quantities in fossil fuels, minerals and rocks and is therefore emitted during the combustion of coal, oil or fossil-fuel gas, the production of cement, and from metallurgical processes. Disposal of sewage sludges, which may contain mercury arising principally from industrial losses, also releases mercury to the environment.

11. The chloralkali industry was responsible in 1975 for emissions of about 18 tonnes of mercury to water, about 22 tonnes to the atmosphere (4 tonnes of which were in hydrogen gas burnt as a fuel), 1·4 tonnes in the caustic soda produced, and 73 tonnes in waste sludges. It was unable to account for 167 tonnes of mercury.

12. All the mercury in paint and adhesives can be considered as released into some part of the environment. The same may be true of the mercury used in catalysis and pharmaceuticals, but the quantity actually released from electrical applications and thermometers etc. is unknown.

13. The agricultural and related uses of mercury are primarily for cereal seed and sugar beet seed treatment, for control of diseases in brassicae, onions and sports turf, for treatment of fruit trees and for dipping seed potatoes and bulbs. Clearly, all of this mercury is irreversibly released into various parts of the environment and this has led to much investigation. What is important here is the extent to which these practices result, if at all, in enhanced availability of mercury to plants, animals or man. In general, the effect of the agricultural use of mercury is very small. Thus cereal seeds treated with mercury produce harvested grain containing only very small quantities of mercury ($\dagger$ < 0·1 ppm*); the spraying of fruit trees produces fruit with mean levels (<0·07 ppm) not very different from levels in unsprayed fruit (ca 0·005–0·04 ppm); and most crops grown on land treated with mercury-containing sewage sludge show only a minimal uptake of the additional mercury into their edible parts, even when mercury levels in the soil are 100 times the normal levels.

$\dagger$ < means less than.
*1 ppm is one part per million.

4

14. The use of mercury in dental fillings presents no hazard to the patient, but dental staff may be at risk from airborne mercury. This is dealt with in Chapter 3.

15. Combustion of coal possibly releases about 12–36 tonnes of mercury to air annually in the UK. This probably becomes widely dispersed and diluted. Oil combustion probably releases about 5 tonnes of mercury annually and cement production about 2 tonnes; this mercury is also likely to be widely dispersed, eventually being deposited on the ground or in waters. Combustion of fossil-fuel gas also probably releases a few tonnes of mercury to air each year.

16. Sewage sludges may contain mercury concentrated from industrial (and domestic and agricultural) effluent. Sludges are disposed of by dumping at sea, by landfill or incineration or are used as fertilisers. About 10 tonnes of mercury enter the sea annually around England and Wales as a consequence of sludge dumping from ships. The total quantity of mercury in sludges disposed of each year by landfill, incineration and use as fertiliser is also probably about 10 tonnes.

17. Non-ferrous metal ores almost invariably contain traces of mercury. Processing releases part of the mercury content to the atmosphere and this may total up to about 5 tonnes annually in the UK. Iron and steel production similarly release only a few tonnes of mercury annually.

18. World-wide, man's activities possibly release up to about 5,000 tonnes of mercury annually; this is clearly much smaller than the estimated global natural mobilisation of 150,000 tonnes per year. However, the significance of man's emissions is that they are often localised and may therefore give rise to enhanced concentrations in certain parts of the environment which represent pathways by which mercury can reach animals and man.

Concentrations in the Environment

The atmosphere

19. Naturally occurring concentrations of mercury vapour in air vary very widely, from <1 ng/m³* in remote areas and over the seas to tens of thousands of ng/m³ near ore deposits and in areas of volcanic activity. For urban areas of the UK what little data there are indicate that average concentrations of mercury vapour range from <100 ng/m³ away from known major sources to about 1,000 ng/m³ within a few hundred metres of a very large chloralkali works†. In rural areas of the UK, concentrations of airborne particulate mercury (i.e. present as airborne dusts) range from 0·04–0·20 ng/m³. There are as yet very few data for such mercury in many urban areas of the UK, but in the

---

*1 ng/m³ is 1 nanogram (thousand-millionth part of a gram) per cubic metre of air.
†The Environmental Protection Agency of the United States of America has recently proposed that 'an ambient air mercury concentration of 1 µg/m³ (= 1000 ng/m³) averaged over a 30 day period will protect the public health with an ample margin of safety'. (Federal Register, Tuesday, 14 October 1975. Vol. 40, No 199, p 48297.)

Swansea Valley, maximum concentrations of 1–14 ng/m³ have been measured. In mainland European conurbations, mean concentrations of about 3 ng/m³, with peak levels up to 15 ng/m³, have been observed.

The hydrosphere

20. Mercury concentrations in rainwater in rural areas of the UK are <0·0002 ppm. There are very few data on drinking water, groundwaters or street surface run-off waters. River waters usually have very low concentrations of mercury, in uncontaminated areas concentrations are usually <0·00005 ppm. Major rivers into which industrial discharges are made may have more than 0·001 ppm. Estuarine and marine waters have mercury levels ranging from 0·00001– 0·00025 ppm, depending on the degree of contamination, which arises principally from industrial and sewage effluent and sewage sludge disposal.

The lithosphere

21. The lithosphere comprises all crustal materials such as rocks, soils and sediments. The concentration of inorganic mercury in soils of the UK is usually <0·1 ppm although higher concentrations do occur, especially in naturally-mineralised areas and where inorganic mercury has been applied consistently to the soil over a fairly long period either in fungicides or in sewage sludges.

22. Concentrations in rocks in general in the UK are similarly low, usually being <0·1 ppm with an average of about 0·07 ppm, but in particular mineral deposits, concentrations of mercury can range up to about 47 ppm; however, there are no known exploitable mercury deposits in the UK.

23. Sediments may contain widely varying concentrations of mercury, arising both from natural causes and the influence of mercury-using industries. In unpolluted areas, river sediments usually have <0·1 ppm mercury, but downstream of mercury discharge points much higher levels are observed. Sediments from major rivers to which industrial discharges are made likewise may contain high concentrations (Table 3). Sediments from tidal and estuarine regions, if free from man-made pollution, usually contain <0·1 ppm mercury but locally much higher concentrations may exist. Marine sediments are comparable, with unpolluted levels of <0·1 ppm and higher levels in polluted areas. In the extreme case of Minamata Bay, Japan, concentrations of 800 ppm were observed.

24. In both the freshwater and marine situation, higher mercury levels have been observed in the surface sediments. This is usually attributed to the influence of man's industrial activities, but the extent to which natural processes might lead to this phenomenon is uncertain.

25. The importance of mercury in sediments lies in the fact that all forms of mercury therein may be converted by natural processes to the more toxic methylmercury compounds. Although de-methylation processes also occur, methyl compounds can be accumulated and concentrated in aquatic organisms and thus may find their way to man via fish and shellfish foods. However, it

must be recognised that mercury contained in sediments which are not in contact with food chains, and which can be maintained out of such contact, is in effect immobilised.

The biosphere

26. *Plants.* It is not certain what proportion of the mercury content of soils can be absorbed by plants and translocated to the edible parts. However, mercury concentrations in plants grown on agricultural soils usually range from about $0 \cdot 001-0 \cdot 2$ ppm, with mean values of about $0 \cdot 01-0 \cdot 04$ ppm (wet weight). Even when grown on soils containing relatively high concentrations of mercury derived from, e.g. sewage sludge, plants usually take up only a very small proportion of the additional mercury. The fate of mercury compounds used in agriculture and their influence on residues in food crops is discussed in detail in Appendix I, and the foods forming part of man's diet are considered in Chapter 2.

27. Aquatic vegetation usually contains much more mercury than the water in which it grows; even so, levels in plants in unpolluted waters are typically in the range $0 \cdot 03-0 \cdot 08$ ppm. Downstream from mercury discharges, much higher levels, e.g. up to 37 ppm, have been observed. Even very low concentrations of mercury in water, e.g. $0 \cdot 00006$ ppm, are reported to inhibit the growth of some species of phytoplankton.

28. *Animals.* Mercury can be transported through food chains firstly by uptake from water or sediment by bacteria, phytoplankton etc. and subsequently by one species feeding on another. The greatest concentration occurs at the first step and zooplankton in unpolluted areas typically have concentrations of about $0 \cdot 14$ ppm mercury compared with $0 \cdot 00003$ ppm in the water. Freshwater fish and shellfish living in unpolluted areas typically have mercury concentrations $<0 \cdot 2$ ppm (wet weight) and this is not significantly different from levels observed 40 years ago. However, in contaminated waters, e.g. downstream from a chloralkali plant, higher levels up to several ppm have been observed. In the exceptional case of the Agano River in Niigata, Japan, where the second outbreak of Minamata disease occurred, levels in fish were up to 23 ppm.

29. Even in waters unpolluted by man, certain fish (e.g. bass, pike) may contain of the order of $0 \cdot 5$ ppm mercury (wet weight) and here it has been noted that concentrations increase with increasing age (or size) of the fish.

30. The situation for marine fish and shellfish is similar. On a wet weight basis, the typical range for fish from unpolluted areas is $0 \cdot 01-0 \cdot 3$ ppm (with means of ca $0 \cdot 05-0 \cdot 01$ ppm), whereas in areas known to be polluted, e.g. certain coastal waters of the UK, levels in individual fish up to $2 \cdot 5$ ppm have been observed, although the mean here is usually $<0 \cdot 5$ ppm. Fish forming part of the UK diet are considered in Chapter 2. In Minamata Bay, fish contained up to 50 ppm mercury.

31. Certain fish such as tuna, halibut or marlin may contain more mercury

than other fish even in apparently unpolluted waters. By examining specimens from museums, attempts have been made to determine whether this is a natural phenomenon, but the uncertainties associated with the purity of preservation materials and with the influence of time on concentrations are yet to be resolved.

32. The most important feature of mercury in fish is that the great majority of it, ca 90 per cent, is usually present in the form of methylmercury compounds.

33. There is also a considerable amount of data on mercury levels in birds. Residues in fish-eating predators in Sweden were one of the first warnings of the influence of mercury-using industries on wildlife and following restrictions in usage, there has been some evidence of decreasing mercury levels in wildlife. Concentrations of mercury are highest in the liver and for British coastal sea birds such as puffins, guillemots and gannets have on occasion ranged from 5–50 ppm (dry weight) and exceptionally of the order of 100 ppm (dry weight). Levels in the eggs of such species are typically 1–6 ppm (dry weight). In exceptional cases, mercury could have contributed to death and it has been suggested that wading birds feeding in polluted estuaries may be at risk. Wild birds such as wood-pigeons, which are occasionally used for human consumption, and some game birds have on occasion been found to contain higher than normal levels of mercury in their livers (up to ca 10 ppm, wet weight). The excessive mortality of these birds was attributed to unusually easy access to, and consumption of, cereal seeds treated with mercury and the insecticide dieldrin. The cause of death has generally been considered to be the insecticide rather than the mercury compounds. The bodies of these birds, and also of living field mice which have fed upon the seed, form obvious sources of mercury to predatory mammals and birds.

CHAPTER 2

PATHWAYS OF MERCURY TO MAN

34. In this Chapter the various ways in which mercury reaches man are described. For the great majority of the general public, the most important site of entry of mercury compounds, particularly methylmercury, to the body is the alimentary tract. Absorption via the respiratory tract is usually of only minor or negligible importance, except for those occupationally exposed; such people may also absorb significant amounts of mercury through the skin.

Food

35. Mercury can get into food for human consumption in a wide variety of ways, both from natural and industrial or agricultural sources, but these are not all of equal significance. The *possible* routes include:

1. via fish and shellfish which take in mercury from the water, sediments or food organisms: this mercury may be of natural origin or due to man's activities; 80–90 per cent of mercury in fish is usually in the methyl form and fish are therefore important when considering the pathways of mercury to man;

2. via meat-producing animals by:
2.1 consumption of herbage which itself has a small natural mercury content derived from the soil and which may also be contaminated by aerial deposition of mercury or by the spraying or spreading of mercury-containing sewage sludges;
2.2 consumption of animal feeds which contain mercury derived from the fish forming the basis of the feedstuff;
2.3 consumption of mercury-treated seeds by wild birds such as wood pigeons, which are occasionally used for human consumption, and game birds;
2.4 inhalation of airborne mercury (likely to be of negligible importance);
2.5 ingestion of mercury-contaminated water (likely to be of negligible importance).

3. via plants by:
3.1 uptake of mercury from the soil: this is largely derived from that naturally present in the soil, but other possibilities include uptake from soils contaminated with mercury by deposition from the air, by use of mercurial dressings or mercury-contaminated sewage sludge as fertilisers; very little is likely to be in the methyl form and uptake is usually minimal;
3.2 contamination of outer surfaces of plants by deposition of airborne

9

particulate mercury in the vicinity of emission sources, e.g. coal-burning installations;

3.3 transfer of mercurial seed-treatments or fruit sprays to the edible part of the plant: this occurs only to an extremely small extent.

Other possible but exceptional routes involving the alimentary tract include:

4. aerial contamination by elemental or particulate mercury of prepared foodstuffs, e.g. foods consumed in contaminated factory areas;

5. misuse in the production of human foodstuffs of mercury-treated seeds originally intended for sowing, or misuse of such seeds as animal feed, the animal subsequently being consumed; both may involve alkylmercury compounds;

6. accidental ingestion of mercury-containing products other than food.

36. It is not possible to assess quantitatively the importance of all of these possibilities. However, it is clear from a comparison of the contributions each makes to the total diet that fish and shellfish account for about half the average daily mercury intake in the UK, whilst fresh meats and dairy products, vegetables and cereals are comparatively minor sources. It should be noted that ingestion via routes 3.2 and 4 can be reduced by discarding the outer leaves of items such as green vegetables, and then washing the foodstuffs before cooking; in the industrial situation, it is important to ensure that the storage of food and consumption occur only in uncontaminated atmospheres. Route 5, as mentioned earlier, has been a cause of major poisoning incidents in some countries, and these arose due to inadequate labelling or marking or deliberate misuse. There have been isolated incidents in the UK in which properly labelled mercury treated seed had been fed to cattle and hens, but action by the authorities prevented any risk of harm to people arising through the consumption of contaminated eggs, meat or milk.

The aquatic path

37. The importance and significance of this route or web of routes is outlined at paragraph 25. Briefly, the important factors are biotransformation of mercury in sediments to methylmercury compounds, concentration and accumulation by aquatic organisms, and ready absorption by man, with only very slow excretion. (In nature, there is also breakdown of organomercury compounds to less toxic forms (paragraph A23).) Accumulation of mercury by living things may occur by direct assimilation, or by passage through a number of steps in a food chain. The basic food materials in water are dissolved substances or insoluble substances that can be converted to the needs of the organism. Phytoplankton and the higher plants are the principal organisms of conversion. In freshwater, a typical food chain might involve zooplankton, insects, snails and small fish feeding on phytoplankton and plants, and then larger fish feeding in turn on the zooplankton, insects, snails and small fish. In the marine environment, insects are of no significance and pelagic fish feed only on zooplankton and smaller fish. Once mercury is introduced at the beginning of a food chain, it may become available to all organisms in the chain. Accumulation occurs when

the rate of intake by an organism exceeds the rate of excretion and levels in predators are often higher than in their prey. The accumulation of relatively high levels (i.e. greater than about 0·5 ppm) is a phenomenon that is associated not solely with fish living in waters contaminated by man's activities; it also occurs quite naturally even in waters having low natural levels of mercury. As far as man's diet is concerned, the higher levels are of significance in only a few types of fish, particularly tuna. Concentrations of mercury in particular fish and shellfish which form part of the UK diet have been reported in detail (HMSO, 1971; HMSO, 1973a) and a summary of the findings is given later in this Chapter.

The terrestrial path

38. These routes include animal and plant foods eaten by man. Animals grazing on herbage ingest the natural mercury content of that herbage (usually a few thousandths of a ppm). Animals also eat feedstuffs prepared from vegetable matter such as groundnuts, soya-beans and grain, and from animal matter such as fish, milk and meat and bone. Concentrations of mercury in such feeds have been reported previously (HMSO, 1971). Feeds prepared from vegetable matter contained levels of <0·01–0·07 ppm, from fish <0·01–1·8 ppm (although the majority of these contained <0·3 ppm), from milk 0·01 ppm and from meat and bone usually 0·01–4 ppm, although one of these samples contained 9·1 ppm. Mean levels were 0·01–0·04 ppm (vegetable feeds), 0·06–0·23 ppm (fish feeds) and 0·37 ppm (meat and bone meal). It seems reasonable to conclude that natural herbage and vegetable-based feeds are of little significance as a source of mercury in animals, that fish meal may be more important (depending on how much is eaten), especially in view of the fact that the mercury content is likely to be largely in the methylated form, and that meat and bone meal may also be important, although here only a negligible proportion of the mercury is present as methylmercury compounds. A small proportion of the mercury ingested by animals is absorbed and this appears mainly in the liver and kidneys, with much less in muscle tissues. Typical values are given later for samples of the UK diet.

39. Game birds such as pheasants and wild birds such as wood pigeons are eaten by man and very occasionally may contain appreciable quantities of mercury derived from seeds treated with mercury. In East Lothian, following a period of difficult sowing conditions and consequent undue access of wildlife to the seeds, mercury levels in the breast tissues of wood pigeons were found to be in the range 0·06–1·22 ppm, with a mean of 0·43 ppm. This occurred in the spring of 1973, but concentrations fell to the usual level of <0·01–0·18 ppm (mean 0·03 ppm) by the summer of the same year. The majority of such mercury is likely to be in the organic form, though not necessarily as methylmercury compounds. It may be calculated that, on a local scale and for restricted periods of time (i.e. about 2 months following sowing), consumption of 0·7 kg (about 1·5 lb) of pigeon flesh per week would lead to the WHO provisional tolerable weekly intake for mercury (paragraph 48) being exceeded. However, in the long term (e.g. a period of 2 years), mean concentrations of mercury in

pigeon flesh are such that a weekly consumption of 3 kg (7 lb) would be required for the WHO tolerable intake to be exceeded: clearly this is very unlikely to occur.

40. Uptake of mercury from the soil by plants is considered in paragraph A72 of Appendix I. Only limited uptake to the edible parts of crops occurs whether the plant is grown on uncontaminated soils or on soils treated with mercury-contaminated sewage sludge. Translocation of mercury seed treatments from the seed to the grain occurs to such a limited extent that it is difficult to demonstrate; this is consistent with the low level of mercury in UK cereal crops.

Mercury in the UK diet

41. Following reports from the USA in 1970 that high levels of methylmercury had been found in canned tuna, a monitoring programme for heavy metals in food was expanded under the control of the Ministry of Agriculture, Fisheries and Food (MAFF). As part of the programme, over 6,400 samples of food were analysed, the results of which were published in two Reports (HMSO, 1971; 1973a).

42. The results in the two Reports are similar. Generally, the mean level of mercury found in cereals, most fresh meats, fruits and preserves, green and root vegetables was <0·005 ppm (fresh weight). Higher levels were found in a variety of canned fish, e.g. in salmon, herrings, pilchards, sardines and mackerel, where the overall mean value was about 0·02 ppm; in pigs' kidney and liver, for which means of 0·05 ppm and 0·03 ppm respectively were found; in canned tuna, where means of 0·07–0·44 ppm were found in different types; and in canned shellfish, e.g. shrimps, prawns, crab and lobster, where means of 0·01–0·29 ppm were found in samples from different waters.

43. Mercury residues in fish were examined in considerable detail. The level was found to depend upon the area from which the fish were taken and also on the fish specie. The mean mercury content of fish from distant waters was 0·03–0·06 ppm, whilst that for fish from middle-distance waters was 0·11–0·21 ppm: these two categories account for 58 per cent and 16 per cent respectively of the total catch in England and Wales. For fish taken up to 25 miles off the coast, the mean concentration was 0·29 ppm, but varied from area to area (this value was biased by the greater extent of sampling carried out in areas of relatively high concentrations); those from the Thames Estuary and the Eastern Irish Sea contained most at 0·45–0·5 ppm and 0·55–0·64 ppm respectively. Fish from these areas represent less than 1 per cent of the total catch landed in the UK.

44. In 1973 cod, haddock, plaice and herring accounted for 61 per cent of the total UK fish catch. The mean mercury concentrations of these fish were within the range 0·04–0·13 ppm; the estimated overall mean mercury concentration for all fish landed in UK was 0·08 ppm. Certain species such as flounder, bass or mullet contain higher levels of mercury, but these do not form a substantial part of the UK dietary fish intake.

45. The mean mercury content of shellfish from coastal areas around England and Wales was 0·16 ppm, the highest levels again being found in the Eastern Irish Sea. For the UK as a whole, the mean concentration for shellfish was 0·13 ppm; shellfish represent a very minor item in the national diet.

46. The amount of mercury in freshwater fish varied from 0·01 ppm in freshwater trout to 1·6 ppm in pike. Abnormally high levels were found in trout and eels in a small river in eastern Scotland, the mean values being 0·08 ppm in trout and 5·8 ppm in eels. Unsatisfactory effluent control at a seed potato treatment plant using an organomercury fungicide was responsible and effluent discharges from the plant were immediately stopped pending the installation of a satisfactory method of waste treatment and disposal. As a precautionary measure, restrictions on fishing in the area were imposed for a short period although there was no evidence of actual harm to health from consumption of fish.

47. Analyses of fish for organic mercury compounds showed that usually about 90 per cent of the total mercury was present in the methyl form. For shellfish the proportion was rather variable, 40–90 per cent being present as methylmercury.

48. The estimated range for the total dietary intake of mercury arising out of the 1·5 kg of food eaten daily by the average individual in the UK is 5–10 μg†/ day, the contribution from fish being about 2–5 μg. This total intake is not significantly different from the average daily intake of less than 14 μg estimated from total diet studies for 1966–67 (Abbott and Tatton, 1970) or from the 5–20 μg estimated in 1949 (Monier-Williams, 1949). This consistency over such lengthy time intervals is reassuring. Furthermore, the intake is substantially lower than the figure proposed by a joint Food and Agriculture Organisation/ World Health Organisation Expert Committee (WHO, 1972a) as a provisional tolerable weekly intake from food; this was given as 0·3 mg*/person/week, of which not more than 0·2 mg should be methylmercury, i.e. about 43 μg/day, of which not more than ca 30 μg should be methylmercury.

49. The amount of mercury ingested varies from day to day and from one person to another because mercury levels in different sorts of food and in different samples of the same type of food, and people's eating habits, vary widely. The probability that *all* foods in a normal mixed diet will consistently have high mercury contents over long periods of time (weeks or months) is extremely low. However, in one case where a few people eating large amounts of fish taken from certain areas and containing higher than average amounts of mercury were studied (HMSO, 1971), higher than average levels of mercury in the blood were found (about 0·015 ppm by weight compared with an average of about 0·005 ppm). This level constitutes no hazard to health, being only marginally higher than levels usually observed (0·005–0·010 ppm) for those not occupationally exposed to mercury (Dinman and Hecker, 1972).

---

†1 μg is 1 microgram (millionth part of a gram) = 1/1000 mg* (milligram, thousandth part of a gram).

13

Drink

50. Drinking water usually contains low concentrations of mercury. Although data for the UK are sparse, those which are available for Europe in general (Table 2) indicate that levels are almost invariably <0·001 ppm (= 0·001 mg/l*), and usually very much lower than this. The situation is similar in the USA (Hammerston et al, 1972). Unpublished data on UK river waters which are used or might be used for the public supply have been obtained in a co-operative survey between some river authorities and the Department of the Environment. This showed that in 80 per cent of cases, *total* mercury concentrations (i.e. including that associated with suspended solids) were <0·001 ppm; in 17 per cent of the cases, levels were in the range 0·001–0·005 ppm; 2 per cent had levels in the range 0·005–0·01 ppm; and 1 per cent had levels of up to 0·05 ppm. The higher concentrations were attributable to point sources of mercury emission, usually industrial in origin. It must be emphasised that the levels quoted here are of *total* mercury and that this metal is usually preferentially adsorbed on solids; treatment of these waters for use as drinking water would remove insoluble mercury.

51. The World Health Organisation has proposed an upper limit for mercury concentrations in drinking water of 0·001 mg/l, or 0·001 ppm by weight. A daily intake of 2 litres of water and water-based beverages with mercury at this level would result in a mercury intake of 0·002 mg/day or 2 μg/day. Even this amount is small compared with the intake from foods; the amount derived from water at the usually-observed concentration of 0·00001–0·00005 ppm (Table 2) is insignificant.

Absorption in the alimentary tract

52. Not more than 0·01 per cent of metallic mercury is absorbed by the alimentary tract. Inorganic mercury salts are absorbed to a greater extent; in human volunteers 15 per cent of a dose was absorbed and this proportion was independent of whether this was protein-bound or not (Clarkson, 1972). The absorption of organic mercury compounds is greater still, but quantitative data for humans are available only for methylmercury, which when given in small quantities is almost completely absorbed from the gastrointestinal tract (Clarkson, 1972).

53. The amount of mercury ingested by the average individual in the UK is about 5–10 μg/day, of which 2–5 μg are in the methylated form. The quantity actually absorbed, if the absorption rates given in the above paragraph apply to the forms of mercury present in food, would be about 2–7 μg/day, of which 2–5 μg may be in the form of methylmercury compounds.

Respiration

54. Mercury vapour and mercury present in airborne dusts may be inhaled; unfortunately, data on which conclusions may be based are sparse. However,

---

*1 mg/l is 1 milligram per litre.

it is reasonable to assume that atmospheric concentrations of mercury vapour in rural areas are likely to be very low (i.e. <1 ng/m³). Average concentrations in some urban areas have been found to be higher, up to about 1,000 ng/m³ within a few hundred metres of a very large chloralkali works. Concentrations of airborne mercury particulates in rural areas of the UK range from $0 \cdot 04$–$0 \cdot 20$ ng/m³, and in urban areas up to about 14 ng/m³. In large mainland European cities, a mean level of about 3 ng/m³, with peaks up to ca 15 ng/m³, has been observed.

55. In the absence of detailed quantitative information on the physical nature of atmospheric particulate mercury and on inhalation, deposition, retention and absorption characteristics, it is not possible to calculate the likely range of daily particulate mercury intakes from respired air. However, even if *all* atmospheric particulate mercury entering the nose and mouth were absorbed during respiration (and this is extremely unlikely) the intake for the general public would still be many times lower than the present average dietary intake in the UK.

56. Mercury vapour entering the alveolar space is almost completely absorbed, so approximately 80 per cent of that inhaled is likely to be absorbed (Kudsk, 1965 and 1969). This means that for those living within a few hundred metres of very large chloralkali works, the average daily absorption via respiration (assuming that an adult breaths about 15 m³ of air each day) could be about 12 μg; (for those living in urban areas with no such local major source, the amount absorbed would be many times lower). Clearly, for those living very near local sources of mercury vapour, respiration can lead to an intake which is comparable in magnitude with dietary intakes. However, it should be noted that the former mercury is almost entirely in the elemental form.

57. Those working in mercury-using industries or in other occupations with exposure to mercury have an enhanced exposure consisting of their uptake from food and the ambient atmosphere, together with uptake from their occupational environment. The significance of occupational exposure is discussed in Chapter 3.

Absorption through the skin

58. In the past, treatment of certain diseases, in particular syphilis, included the application of mercurial ointments to the skin. In some instances the persons applying the ointment excessively increased their body burdens of mercury by skin absorption. This type of therapy is not now employed in the UK. However, some skin-lightening creams, which may contain 10–15 per cent by weight of aminomercuric chloride, are still widely used in some other countries (Barr et al, 1973), and have caused kidney damage (Kibukamusoke et al, 1974). Absorption through the skin in the field of occupational health is discussed in Chapter 3.

CHAPTER 3

MERCURY IN MAN

59. The various pathways by which mercury enters the human body have been described in the previous chapter. This chapter describes the distribution and deposition of mercury in man, the ways in which mercury is excreted from the body, the types of poisoning which exist and industrial experience within the UK.

Distribution, deposition and excretion

60. More than $99 \cdot 9$ per cent of ingested elemental mercury and about 85–97 per cent of ingested inorganic compounds of mercury are excreted within a few days, mainly in the faeces; only a small proportion is actually absorbed into the body tissues. In contrast, the majority (ca 95 per cent) of methylmercury compounds ingested with food is absorbed. Of the mercury vapour entering the lungs, about 80 per cent may be absorbed.

61. After absorption, elemental mercury is partly distributed in this form and oxidised in the tissues, partly oxidised in the blood, and distributed like inorganic mercuric mercury (Magos, 1968). Mercurous compounds, which are practically insoluble, before being absorbed must be decomposed to elemental mercury or oxidised to mercuric mercury, and are then distributed accordingly. Mercuric mercury forms soluble compounds with blood which are associated mainly with the plasma or diffusible thiol compounds and are transported in this form. They are also found in association with other soft tissues, fluids and proteins.

62. Some organic mercury compounds, in particular the phenyl and alkoxyalkyl derivatives, are rapidly converted to the inorganic form, mainly by the liver, and this then behaves like that ingested in an inorganic state. The conversion of ethylmercury to the inorganic form is slow and that of methylmercury even slower. These compounds are retained for longer periods in the blood where they are associated primarily with the red blood cells. They penetrate the blood/brain barrier relatively easily and their biological half-life is longer because of their higher affinity for proteins with sulphur-containing groups, because their uptake by the kidneys and urinary excretion is very much less and because after excretion in bile into the intestine a higher proportion is re-absorbed.

63. Once in the body, all forms of mercury become widely distributed in tissues, the greatest accumulation occurring in the kidney and liver. Alkylmercury compounds and elemental mercury also enter the brain tissue, from which they are only slowly eliminated. Recent work on autopsy material (Kosta et al, 1975),

has demonstrated high levels of mercury in thyroid and pituitary tissues of those previously occupationally exposed to elemental mercury. This and other work (Rossi et al, 1976) has shown that selenium is co-accumulated with mercury, and it may be that this is an autoprotective mechanism.

64. Mercury is excreted in the mercuric form after exposure to elemental, inorganic and aryl or alkoxyalkyl mercury. Excretion occurs mainly in the urine and faeces but some is excreted in sweat and saliva. Alkylmercury compounds are excreted slowly: the half-life of methylmercury compounds in man has been estimated as 70–80 days (Aberg et al, 1969; Miettinen et al, 1971). Deposition of mercury occurs in the hair, nails and in the epidermis. Methylmercury (Suzuki et al, 1967; Childs, 1973) and elemental mercury are transferred to the foetus through the placenta (Clarkson et al, 1972; Greenwood et al, 1972); all forms may reach infants via breast milk.

65. Mercury is not known to be essential for the well being of man and the suggestion (Goldwater, 1971) that man may have become dependent on traces of it, following exposure over evolutionary periods of time, is speculative. Mercury compounds have a high affinity for sulphydryl groups, predominantly found in proteins, and they are therefore potent, non-specific enzyme poisons. However, the precise mechanisms of toxicity are not clear. There is evidence (Skerfving et al, 1970) of increased chromosome breakage in blood cells from individuals having a high mercury blood level, but the significance of this remains uncertain. It has long been known that mercury can damage the kidneys; people with renal disorders may therefore be a high risk group if they are subjected to a significant uptake of mercury from any source.

Types of poisoning and associated symptoms

66. Metallic mercury, inorganic salts and organic mercury compounds behave differently in the body. All forms of mercury accumulate in the liver and kidneys, and affect these organs adversely, whereas elemental and alkylmercury compounds also enter the brain.

67. *Acute* poisoning describes the results of an exposure to a single massive dose of a compound, or to multiple exposures over a short period. Acute poisoning has been known to occur on rare occasions in the industrial setting following inhalation of air with mercury concentrations in excess of ca. 1200 $\mu g/m^3$. Such exposures lead to a metallic taste in the mouth, gastro-intestinal symptoms, headache and sometimes albuminuria, followed after a few days by swelling of the salivary glands, ulceration of the mouth and the formation of a dark line on the gums. Later, teeth may be lost. Ingestion of inorganic mercury salts, especially 'sublimate' – once a common method of suicide – is uncommon now. Acute intoxication is characterised by pharyngitis, abdominal pain and vomiting, bloody diarrhoea and shock, but the most characteristic effect is the so-called 'sublimate nephrosis' which depending on its severity, results in oliguria, anuria or death. Acute poisoning by organic mercury compounds is also known. The effects vary with the substance, but skin reactions, followed

17

by blister formation, inflammation of the mouth and throat, myalgia and transient albuminuria have been described. The physical changes and mental deterioration may remain after acute symptoms have disappeared.

68. *Chronic* poisoning results from exposure to small amounts of mercury over a long period of time, and has been known to occur by inhalation of mercury vapour in those working with electrical and other apparatus containing mercury and from contact with inorganic mercury compounds. The nervous system is primarily affected with metallic and organic mercury. Three main groups of symptoms may occur separately or together in varying degrees. These are exaggerated emotional responses (such as timidity, resentfulness, depression, irritability, extreme embarrassment, lack of concentration and poor memory), gingivitis and muscle tremors. Mild cases may exhibit some personality changes, anxiety, insomnia and lack of appetite. Tremors can vary from slight effects on hands, eyelids and the tongue to stammering, difficulty in swallowing and gross inco-ordination. Impaired hearing and inability to communicate may follow. Sensory disturbances, impairment of taste and smell and severe salivation may also occur, as may chronic nasal catarrh with nose-bleeding, renal disease and ocular lesions. A greyish-brown discolouration of the anterior capsule of the eye (mercurialentis) may be seen long after the end of exposure or recovery from chronic poisoning.

69. Another manifestation of chronic poisoning, now only of historical interest, was seen in infants. During the 1950's the condition known as 'Pink Disease' (acrodynia) which had been first described in 1890, was found to be due to the use of mercury-containing teething powders, dusting powders and ointments for children. Poisoned children were often miserable, difficult to placate and apathetic in play. The symptoms were a generalised rash, looking in the first instance like German Measles, and as its most characteristic feature, swollen and painful dusky-pink hands and feet. The extremities were cold and clammy and repeated loss of skin could occur. There was usually no fever, except when the condition was complicated by respiratory infections. Nevertheless there was profuse sweating, encouraging the development of skin infections. An intense dislike of light was not uncommon and extreme muscle weakness and laxity of ligaments were characteristic. Loss of seemingly sound teeth could occur. The normal course of events was for the rash to spread for about a month, the swelling with irritation of the hands or feet to persist for about another month and a slow subsidence over a period of several months. In severe cases, inflamed and swollen gums, accompanied by profuse salivation, progressed to necrosis of the jaw and gangrene could develop. Over the years, many fatalities occurred but since the recognition of the cause it is no longer seen, the use of mercury in this type of product having ceased.

Alkylmercury poisoning

70. Methylmercury compounds have been principally involved here. The methyl form was discharged into the waters of Minamata Bay and gave rise to the Minamata incident (Takeuchi, 1972b). Methylmercury compounds used as

seed-treatments have, as a result of misuse of treated seeds, caused mass poisoning in Iraq (Bakir et al, 1973). Ethylmercury treated grain has caused similar incidents.

71. As mentioned previously, if taken in large enough quantities, there is a considerable risk of accumulation of methylmercury in the body. In severe intoxication permanent organic changes in the brain are seen; these are in contrast to the reversible disturbances usually associated with other forms of chronic mercury poisoning. In chronic methylmercury poisoning constriction of the field of vision amounting to 'tunnel vision', impairment of hearing, disturbances of speech, numbness and tingling of the lips, hand or feet may be seen. Motor changes such as tremors and loss of co-ordination of movement may occur. Involvement of the skin and mucous membrane of the nose and throat may be seen. These symptoms are commonly described as 'Minamata Disease'.

72. Methylmercury can lead to poisoning in the foetus, with damage to the central nervous system. Children exposed in this way may show mental retardation, cerebral palsy and convulsions. Information from Minamata indicates that cytogenic effects occur in the early stages of development and it is possible that these may result from induced chromosomal alterations.

Alkoxyalkylmercury poisoning

73. There have been few cases from exposure to these compounds. Symptoms have included loss of appetite, diarrhoea, weight loss and fatigue. It has not been assessed how far these symptoms might be due to an inorganic mercury compound. Kidney damage has also been reported following excessive exposure to these compounds.

Arylmercury poisoning

74. Very few cases of this type of intoxication have been reported. Irritation of the skin has been described.

Human exposure

75. Mercury concentrations in various human tissues may be considered in the following broad groupings:
    (i) concentrations in tissues of people not occupationally exposed to mercury and eating a normal diet;
    (ii) concentrations in tissues of people not occupationally exposed, but exposed in other ways, e.g. eating a diet with a relatively high mercury content (usually from fish coming from areas of known mercury contamination) or exposed to mercury-containing pharmaceuticals;
    (iii) concentrations in tissues of people occupationally exposed to mercury;
    (iv) concentrations in tissues of people suffering mercury poisoning.

The value of the data is limited, because tissue levels do not always reflect the degree of exposure, particularly at low levels. Nor is there always any correlation

19

between levels in different tissues nor between tissue levels and the onset of clinical symptoms (Harris, 1972). Nevertheless, mercury levels in blood, autopsy or biopsy materials, and urine, can be used to classify the exposure of people on a group basis.

The general public

76. What few data there are for the general public in the UK are reassuring. People coming within the first category have shown blood mercury levels of up to 0·005 ppm and hair levels of 0·8–8·4 ppm (HMSO, 1971). In other countries people in this category have shown blood and hair levels respectively of 0·001–0·02 ppm and 0·1–6 ppm in Finland (Sumari et al, 1972); up to 0·035 ppm and 2–14 ppm in Canada (Mastromatteo and Sutherland, 1972); up to 0·05 ppm, but usually less than 0·003 ppm in blood in 16 different countries (Goldwater, 1965); 0·005–0·028 ppm in blood in the USA (Dinman and Hecker, 1972); 0·005–0·02 ppm in blood of an urban American population and 0·003–0·057 ppm in blood of a Venezuelan Indian tribe (Hecker et al, 1974); 1·9–6·2 ppm in hair in Japan (Ohta, 1966); and 0·1–4 ppm in hair in Iraq (Al-Shahristani and Al-Haddad, 1973). It has been suggested that the 'normal' blood mercury concentration in this group is 0·005–0·010 ppm (Dinman and Hecker, 1972).

77. There have recently been attempts in the USA to establish base-line data for concentrations of mercury in various tissues of the human body for those not occupationally exposed to mercury (Mottet and Body, 1972; Stein et al, 1974). The concentrations did not correlate with age or sex, but the data suggested that urban dwellers had a somewhat greater mercury burden than rural people.

78. In the second group (not occupationally exposed, but having a higher than average consumption of fish with a relatively high mercury content), blood and hair levels in UK subjects were in the ranges 0·010–0·030 ppm and 1·2–3·9 ppm respectively (HMSO, 1971). Higher values have been observed in people in comparable groups from other parts of the world. Thus in the USA, blood levels of 0·007–0·051 ppm have been reported (Wilcox, 1972); in Canada, blood and hair levels of 0·02–0·085 ppm (exceptionally up to 0·155 ppm) and 10–96 ppm respectively have been recorded (Mastromatteo and Sutherland, 1972); in Finland, blood and hair levels of 0·002–0·2 ppm and 0·3–50 ppm respectively have been reported (Sumari et al, 1972); and in Peru, levels of methylmercury in blood of 0·011–0·275 ppm have been observed (Turner et al, 1974).

79. This second group also includes those exposed to mercury through mercury-containing pharmaceuticals. Reference has already been made to Pink Disease. In one examination (Howie and Smith, 1967) analyses were made of the mercury levels in hair and urine from children with this condition. The hair samples proved to be of no value in detecting over-exposure, but excretion of mercury in the urine was high, ranging from 86–859 μg/l before treatment: in comparison,

the upper limit of acceptability widely used in the industrial setting is 300 μg/1. Pink Disease is now only of historical importance but high levels of mercury in hair and fingernails have confirmed that the use of mercury-containing skin-lightening creams continues (Barr et al, 1973b). A group of people exposed in this way had head hair levels of 20–9220 ppm mercury and fingernail levels of 5–840 ppm, compared with levels of 0·5–23·4 ppm mercury and 0·4–22 ppm mercury respectively in a control group which had not used such preparations.

80. Mercury metal and compounds of mercury are used in laboratories of educational establishments under the control of Local Education Authorities and in universities. The main danger in schools arises from inhalation of mercury vapour unless the metal is handled with appropriate care. The Department of Education and Science has issued a safety booklet (DES Safety Booklet No. 2, HMSO, 1976) giving guidance on, amongst other things, precautions to be taken to control possible exposure of pupils and students to mercury vapour following spillage or heating of mercury metal or certain of its compounds. Furthermore, detailed guidance is being considered at present, including the possibility of monitoring laboratory atmospheres for mercury. There is no evidence that this use of mercury and its compounds has led to any undue exposure. The use of mercury and its compounds in university laboratories is not subject to specific controls at present. The Committee of Vice-Chancellors and Principals is preparing a Code of Practice for safety in universities of which Part 1, General Principles, was issued in 1975. Part 2 is intended to cover specific hazards and is at present being considered by this Committee.

Industrial experience

81. The fact that exposure to mercury and its compounds can result in poisoning has been known since classical times. Indeed, almost 2,000 years ago, Pliny the Elder described the sufferings of slaves working in mercury mines. The most important routes of entry for those occupationally exposed are via the lungs and absorption through the skin. Respiratory absorption in the UK largely involves the vapour rather than the particulate form, and absorption through the skin can occur with both the element and its compounds. Studies of industrial workers have often shown a greater degree of mercury absorption (as judged from the concentration of mercury in the urine) than would be expected from the maximum possible inhaled quantity: this indicates the importance of absorption through the skin, and examples of such exposure include those engaged in the manufacture of mercury vapour lamps (Buckell et al, 1946) and dentists, dental staff and dental technicians handling mercury (Lenihan et al, 1973).

82. The hazards associated with the use of mercury amalgams in dentistry have recently been reviewed (Lenihan et al, 1973). During treatment, the patient may ingest or inhale mercury or ingest fragments of filling, but this constitutes no hazard because metallic mercury passes through the digestive tract with practically no absorption; amalgam too is almost insoluble in saliva and gastric juices. Moreover, the patient is unlikely to be exposed for more than a few days

per year. Although higher than usual amounts of mercury are excreted following insertion of fillings this may be due to inhalation of mercury at the surgery rather than leaching from the filling and the Chief Medical Officer of the Department of Health and Social Security concluded in 1971 that there was no evidence of any harm occurring.

83. There may be more serious hazards for those working in dental practices and in particular for those handling mercury, since they may be exposed for much of their working life. Atmospheric mercury levels in 23 surgeries were found (Lenihan et al, 1973) to vary from <10 $\mu g/m^3$* to 70 $\mu g/m^3$ for the vapour, but from 25 $\mu g/m^3$ to 800 $\mu g/m^3$ for total mercury, i.e. including the particulates. The accepted limit for occupational exposure is 50 $\mu g/m^3$ over a 40 hour working week (see paragraph 88). It is therefore not surprising that dentists and surgery assistants had higher levels of mercury in hair and nails than other staff not handling mercury; one death has been claimed (Cook et al, 1969). American experience (Gronka et al, 1970; Cuzacq et al, 1971; Miller et al, 1974) is similar to the UK experience. However, the British Dental Association has, through its journal and by direct contact with its members, issued advice on procedures to be adopted to reduce to a minimum exposure in the surgery. And in the UK, the health of all workers, including the self-employed, is safeguarded by the Health and Safety at Work etc. Act 1974, which is administered by the Health and Safety Executive.

84. Acute mercury poisoning is very rare in industry. Chronic poisoning is also uncommon, although an enhanced absorption of mercury can be demonstrated in many workers using mercury. Poisoning by mercury in any form, when it occurs as a result of employment and in a place of employment to which the Factories Act 1961 applies is a condition notifiable to the Chief Inspector of Factories, Health and Safety Executive. The number of cases officially notified annually in the UK has remained between none and six over the last half century. Almost all of these have been due to the metal or to inorganic compounds, and few to organic compounds.

85. In recent years, attention has been increasingly directed to the occasional development of nephrosis with water retention and oedema. However, it is not known with certainty how much more common this condition is among those occupationally exposed than in the general population. The appearance of small to moderate amounts of protein in the urine of mercury workers is not uncommon and, although not usually associated with any clinical symptoms, has on rare occasions occurred before the onset of nephrosis.

86. The compounds which most commonly affect the skin are phenylmercury acetate (a fungicide), which can blister unprotected skin, alkoxyalkylmercury compounds, and mercury fulminate (used in the munitions industry) which has given rise to much dermatitis affecting especially the webs of fingers. Those using mercurial fungicides are instructed in their safe use through the Pesticides Safety Precautions Scheme (see Chapter 4).

---

*1 $\mu g/m^3$ is 1 microgramme per cubic metre of air $= 1000$ ng/m^3.

87. Statutory control of the use of mercury in industry and agriculture to ensure safety is by means of The Health and Safety at Work etc. Act 1974, Section 2, which makes a general requirement for employers to ensure the safety, health and welfare of their employees, and in industry by the Factories Act 1961, Section 63, which requires the control of dust, fumes and other impurities which are likely to be injurious or offensive to the persons employed. These Acts are administered by the Health and Safety Commission through the Health and Safety Executive, which employs HM Inspectors of Factories, who are able to advise on the nature of precautionary measures. Some of this advice is available in published form, e.g. Technical Data Note 21 (revised), "Mercury"; leaflet SHW 337, "Mercurial Poisoning" and Detection of Toxic Substances in Air, Booklet No. 13, "Mercury and Compounds of Mercury".

88. HM Factory Inspectorate, Health and Safety Executive, also publishes a list of threshold limit values (TLVs) for a wide range of toxic substances encountered in industry (HMSO, 1973b). TLVs refer to airborne concentrations and represent conditions to which it is believed nearly all workers may be repeatedly exposed for an 8-hour working day and a 40-hour working week without adverse effects. For metallic mercury and all its compounds other than the alkyl derivatives, the TLV is currently 50 $\mu g/m^3$, with an excursion factor of 3; this means that occasional peaks up to 150 $\mu g/m^3$ are permitted. In the case of alkyl derivatives, a lower TLV of 10 $\mu g/m^3$ with occasional peaks up to 15 $\mu g/m^3$, has been adopted. Metallic mercury vapour levels in the atmosphere can be conveniently monitored by the use of an ultraviolet light spectrophotometer, and such instruments can also be adapted for the measurement of organic mercury compounds.

89. No regulations made under the Factories Act require medical examination of those working with mercury. But, in practice, many such people are screened by the Employment Medical Advisory Service, usually by analysis of urine samples for mercury; in addition, a clinical assessment is made. There is a lack of unanimity on what constitutes an upper limit of acceptability of the concentration of mercury in urine; a figure of 300 $\mu g/l$ has been widely used, but up to 600 $\mu g/l$ has been suggested. There is no clear-cut relationship, in individuals, between the level of mercury in the urine and the presence of symptoms of poisoning. Urinary concentrations as high as 1000 $\mu g/l$ are recorded occasionally in symptom-free workers and nephrosis has appeared in workers in whom excretion has subsequently been found to be low. In the latter case, the possibility that impaired excretion by the damaged kidneys has led to low concentrations of mercury in urine cannot, of course, be excluded. The use of a group moving average has been advocated and is often used as a means of monitoring the working environment.

Hazardous levels

90. Levels of mercury in tissues from subjects in category (iv) of paragraph 75 above vary widely and it is impossible to define precisely the level associated with a particular biochemical effect or with a specific symptom of poisoning.

However, it is clear that tissue mercury levels in cases of poisoning are much higher than those quoted above (paragraphs 76–78) for the general public. In Japan, the mean blood level of those poisoned at Niigata was 1–3 ppm (Dinman and Hecker, 1972) (although the minimum at which signs and symptoms of methylmercury poisoning appeared has been estimated at 0·2 ppm (Berglund et al, 1971)), and their mean hair level was 369 ppm; in the incident in Alamogordo, New Mexico, blood mercury levels in those poisoned by the flesh of hogs fed on mercury treated seeds were probably in the range of 2·9–4·4 ppm (Dinman and Hecker, 1972); in a case of fatal poisoning in Sweden, the blood level was about 4 ppm (Dinman and Hecker, 1972); in the Iraqi incident, involving consumption of bread made from treated seeds, levels in the first samples of blood of those poisoned ranged from 1·1–3·7 ppm (Bakir et al, 1973). Hair levels of 120–600 ppm were associated with mild symptoms of poisoning, 200–800 ppm with moderate symptoms and 400–1,600 ppm with severe symptoms (Al-Shahristani and Al-Haddad, 1973); the minimum blood mercury level associated with signs of poisoning was 0·2 ppm in Iraqi mothers and about 0·55 ppm in infants (Amin-Zaki et al, 1974).

91. It is not known with certainty how much methylmercury must be ingested to precipitate symptoms of poisoning in man. However, in Japan, the intake probably averaged about 30 μg/kg body weight/day, over several months, although accurate exposure data were not available (Berglund et al, 1971). For the poisoning epidemic in Iraq, calculations based on information given by the patients on their bread consumption and the use of contaminated flour indicate that a daily intake of 28–44 μg/kg body weight/day over 45 days produced paraesthesia and 56–88 μg/kg body weight/day produced ataxia. The average daily uptake in the New Mexican incident (see paragraph 90 above) was probably in the range 50–60 μg/kg body weight/day. The provisional tolerable weekly intake of mercury from food proposed by the joint FAO/WHO committee is 0·3 mg/person/week, of which not more than 0·2 mg should be in the methylated form. (This is equivalent, for a 70 kg adult, to an intake of about 0·6 μg/kg body weight/day, with not more than 0·4 μg/kg body weight/day in the methyl form.) The WHO limit is thus about 70 times lower than the amount which could induce poisoning. The actual amount of total mercury ingested from food by the average individual in the UK is about 5–10 μg/day (0·035–0·070 mg/week or 0·07–0·14 μg/kg body weight/day for an adult) and only about half of this is in the methylated form; these figures are about 4–8 times lower in terms of total mercury and 6–12 times lower in terms of methylmercury than the WHO provisional tolerable weekly intake.

92. An example may illustrate what these figures mean. In the UK, the average concentration of mercury in fish is 0·08 ppm and it would be necessary for a 70 kg adult to consume about 12·5 kg (27·5 lb) of such fish daily for a period of three months to reach the borderline between toxic and non-toxic body burden. In the case of *continuous daily* consumption, slightly less than 1 kg (2·2 lb) of fish per day would produce a steady-state body burden (when uptake and excretion are in balance) which would still be harmless. In fact,

the average daily consumption of fish in the UK varies from 0·012–0·034 kg per person, or about 0·03–0·08 lb/person/day. Clearly then, there is a large factor of safety here. In relation to the WHO limit of tolerable intake, a *daily* consumption of about 0·5 kg (1·1 lb) of fish with the average mercury concentration would be necessary before the WHO level was exceeded: this level of consumption is still greatly in excess of the UK average. Other countries have deemed it necessary to set a maximum concentration of mercury in fish for human consumption; this is 0·5 ppm (Canada and the USA) and 0·4 ppm (Japan). These limits are based on the WHO provisional tolerable intake and the Japanese figure takes into account their very high fish consumption (a mean of 0·11 kg/day) and low average body weight (50 kg).

93. For the great majority of people in the UK food is the major source of mercury and the average intake is well below the provisional tolerable limit. This is reassuring. However, what is of most importance, particularly to the individual, is the total intake of mercury not only from the diet (which can, in some cases, have a higher than average mercury content) but also from all other sources including e.g. air. Moreover, it is necessary to consider the possible influence of diseases on an individual's tolerance for mercury. While the number of people coming into such categories of special exposure is small and the risk to them is probably low, the possibility must not be dismissed. Since mercury is a hazardous substance playing no known role in human biochemistry or physiology, it is desirable that the total intake from all sources should be kept as low as possible.

C

CHAPTER 4

CONTROLS ON MERCURY, GOVERNMENT ACTION
AND RESEARCH

94. This chapter outlines the fundamental approach to control of pollution adopted in the UK and details how this policy affects the various parts of the environment and the pathways by which mercury may reach man. It thus sets out Government action on mercury in food, on uses of mercury in consumer goods and agriculture, on control of emissions to water and air, on disposal of mercury-containing substances and on research on various aspects of mercury.

Policy

95. In the interests of human health and the protection of man's environment, the UK adopts a comprehensive system of environmental controls involving a 'best practicable means' approach. Underlying this flexible and pragmatic approach is the basic philosophy that the environment can and should be used, but used wisely, and that, to this end, pollution control requirements should be set having regard to, amongst other things, local conditions, technical feasibility and economic desirability as well as the paramount medical and scientific criteria of risk to health or the environment. In short, through controls ranging from outright bans to Codes of Practice, issues are tackled from the point of view of their individual effects on quality objectives set for man and the environment; in this way we seek to avoid the rigidity and consequent misuse of resources associated with unduly legalistic and formalistic procedures. There is no such thing as absolute safety and the objective should be to achieve an acceptable balance between the benefit to be gained by the use of a potentially harmful substance and the risk involved in using it or introducing it to the environment.

Food and drink

96. There are no statutory limits laid down in the UK for the level of mercury residues in food. There are thus no controls that are specifically related to mercury and the only relevant legislation is the general provisions of the Food and Drugs Act 1955. Section 2 of the Act makes it an offence to sell to the purchaser a food which is not of the nature, substance or quality demanded; section 8 makes it an offence to sell food unfit for human consumption. In the case of a dispute, it would ultimately be for the Courts to decide, in the light of all the relevant evidence, whether a particular level of mercury in food rendered it not of the 'nature, substance or quality demanded' or 'unfit for human consumption'. The law is enforced by Food and Drugs authorities and by port health authorities, who have samples of food analysed for, inter alia, their mercury content.

97. The Food Additives and Contaminants Committee, an independent expert body advising Ministers on additives and contaminants, has considered the question of specific statutory limits for mercury on three occasions. The first was in 1970 and concerned only levels of mercury in tuna fish. At that time they endorsed the recommendation of the then Pharmacology Sub-Committee of the Committee on Medical Aspects of Food Policy that there was no need to set a limit on the level of mercury in canned tuna fish. This recommendation took account of the small consumption of tuna in Britain and the results obtained from a limited survey carried out at that time on residue levels in this food.

98. The second occasion was in 1971, prior to publication of the Survey of Mercury in Food, the First Report of the Working Party on the Monitoring of Foodstuffs for Mercury and Other Heavy Metals (HMSO, 1971). The Committee then decided, in the light of the small amounts of mercury detected in the many foods analysed, including fish, that there was no need for statutory residue limits to be imposed. It was felt that until sufficient evidence was available to allow a more accurate assessment of the safe intake level, the satisfactory situation revealed in the above Report should not be upset by imports of fish or any food containing high levels of mercury or methylmercury. They subsequently advised enforcement authorities and public analysts that they could assist in this by constant vigilance, ensuring that food containing levels of mercury unacceptable in their countries of origin did not find their way on to the UK market.

99. The third occasion on which the Committee considered statutory limits was in 1973, prior to publication of Survey of Mercury in Food: A Supplementary Report, the third Report of the Working Party on Monitoring of Foodstuffs for Heavy Metals (HMSO, 1973a). The Committee's views were that statutory limits were not necessary at that time, but that the situation should be kept under review, and that the guidance given to enforcement authorities and public analysts after publication of the first Report should continue to apply.

100. In England and Wales, the regional Water Authorities (and the water companies), which supply water to a wide variety of consumers, have a duty to ensure that water supplied for drinking is 'wholesome': in Scotland, this duty is borne by the Regional Councils and Islands Councils. There are no concentration limits statutorily prescribed for mercury, or indeed for many other substances, and in the event of a dispute it would be for a Court to decide, in the light of the best available evidence, whether water containing a particular level of mercury could be regarded as wholesome. There is already an EEC Directive specifying maximum concentrations for metals, including mercury, in water for abstraction for drinking water production and the limit for mercury is 1 μg/l (0·001 ppm). There is also a draft EEC Directive on water as supplied for human consumption and this will probably prescribe the same maximum concentration for mercury. The WHO have also recommended the same maximum limit for drinking water.

Consumer goods

101. Concentrations of soluble mercury in the dried film of paint, lacquer and varnish coatings on pens, pencils and brushes, and in the cores of such instruments, are limited to 100 ppm by the Pencils and Graphic Instruments (Safety) Regulations 1974, made under the Consumer Protection Act 1961. These regulations came into force on 1 August 1974, and will help to ensure that children do not add significantly to their mercury intake by chewing these items.

102. Paints used on children's toys are also likely to be chewed. These paints are subject to control under the Toys (Safety) Regulations 1974, and these also prescribe a limit of 100 ppm of soluble mercury in the dried film.

103. Some mercurial compounds are included in the Poisons List 1972 (as amended), made under the Pharmacy and Poisons Act 1933. This Act controls the sale and supply of mercurial substances and makes provision for the form of containers for storage and transport and for the labelling of containers with stipulated warnings.

104. An EEC Directive, already in force in the original member states, imposes safety requirements for the classification according to hazard and for the packaging and labelling of dangerous substances, including mercury and its compounds, when these are marketed within the Community. This Directive will take effect in the UK in 1976.

105. There is also a proposal for a directive imposing similar safety requirements, i.e. for classification, packaging and labelling with regard to the marketing of paints, varnishes, adhesives and similar products when these contain more than specified proportions of dangerous substances. Mercury and its compounds are included.

106. There is now an EEC Directive on cosmetics; this excludes elemental mercury and inorganic and organic compounds of mercury from use in cosmetic products, with exemption for two compounds of mercury used as preservatives at low concentrations.

Agricultural uses

107. Since 1957, control has been exercised over the agricultural uses of all forms of mercury pesticides (which includes all fungicides, herbicides etc.) by the Pesticide Safety Precautions Scheme (PSPS). The purpose of this scheme, which is non-statutory (but formally negotiated between Government and industry) and which is operated by MAFF on behalf of the UK agriculture and health departments, is to safeguard humans (whether they be users, consumers of treated produce or other members of the public), livestock, domestic animals and wildlife against risks from pesticides. Under this scheme, anyone wishing to market a pesticide product must provide MAFF with such data as necessary for the Advisory Committee on Pesticides and Other Toxic Chemicals to assess the chemical's safety in use and to make recommendations for safety precautions. Clearance is only granted when the Advisory Committee is satisfied

that it can be safely used and its recommendations appear on the labels of all cleared pesticide products.

108. Under the PSPS, other restrictions can be placed on use. For example, some of the more toxic organomercury seed treatments are restricted to use in premises subject to the Factories Act, because of the operator risks involved. The Scheme also requires manufacturers to supply sack labels for treated seed, carrying warnings to farm workers handling the seed and warnings against use of this seed or sack for food or feed. With only a few exceptions, this has proved satisfactory in eliminating inappropriate use of treated seed in the UK.

109. The EEC are considering possible directives on the safety clearance of pesticides and on the use of organomercurial pesticides in agriculture.

Emissions to air

110. The two most important industrial sources of atmospheric mercury are the chloralkali process and the commercial combustion of fossil fuels. The chloralkali process and the major combustion processes are registered under the Alkali etc. Works Regulation Act and are thus subject in England and Wales to supervision by Her Majesty's Alkali and Clean Air Inspectorate (HMACAI), formerly of the Department of the Environment and now part of the Health and Safety Executive and in Scotland by HM Industrial Pollution Inspectorate (HMIPI). Mercury is scheduled as a noxious or offensive gas under the 1972 Alkali Order for Scotland, although there is no chloralkali industry in Scotland.

111. As mentioned in the Chief Inspector's 109th Annual Report (HMSO' 1972), HMACAI supervise for mercury emissions certain processes used in the production of chlorine. Most attention is being paid to reducing losses arising from purging and venting of dilute hydrogen gas, which contains mercury as an impurity, leaving the 'end-boxes' of the chloralkali cell; this is the largest single source of mercury loss to the atmosphere within this industry. Processes for removing mercury from hydrogen have been developed in recent years, and one is in operation in UK for treatment of mainstream hydrogen from the cells and one for treatment of dilute hydrogen from the end-boxes of cells. Another unit is planned to cover a large chloralkali works and it is intended to extend this control where practicable and necessary. Universal adoption of such treatment processes could probably reduce the overall mercury loss to air within this industry from its present level of about 22 tonnes to about 3–4 tonnes annually, but the need for such measures at individual works, and their practicability, has yet to be established. Most cell rooms are operated with mercury vapour concentrations well below the threshold limit value and further progress in reducing cell room emissions, at least from modern works, is likely to be limited. In cases where higher atmospheric concentrations are found, they can generally be traced to excessive spillage of mercury, often during maintenance operations.

112. HMACAI (and in Scotland HMIPI) also control emissions from the major fuel-consuming industries. Here attention is primarily directed at controlling

particulates, e.g. by the use of electrostatic precipitators at boiler plant using pulverised coal, and ensuring, by the use of tall chimneys, that ground level concentrations of sulphur dioxide are acceptable. Mercury is a trace element in coal, and there is no known practicable method of preventing its emission, during combustion, as a vapour. Losses from power stations are rapidly dispersed and diluted by being exhausted through tall chimneys; losses from the comparable quantity of coal burned domestically in the UK are emitted at much lower level and may thus be less readily dispersed and diluted.

113. As announced previously in Pollution Paper No. 1, "The Monitoring of the Environment in the United Kingdom" (HMSO, 1974a), an Air Pollution Monitoring Management Group has been set up to manage monitoring of air pollution in the UK. A national network of 20 sites, ranging from the urban/industrial to the rural type, has been set up and monitoring for a range of trace elements in air will take place at these sites. Mercury, however, poses special analytical problems because of the need to study both the vapour and particulate forms. Monitoring for mercury is therefore being undertaken at sites of special interest, e.g. around chloralkali works, where concentrations might be expected to be higher than elsewhere. In addition, mercury in rainfall along the east coast of Scotland and England is being monitored as part of a survey of the input of various pollutants to the North Sea.

Emissions to waters

114. Until the provisions of the Control of Pollution Act 1974 have been fully implemented, the legal position with regard to discharges of mercury-containing effluents to mainland waters, estuaries and sewers can be briefly summarised as follows:

(i) all discharges to inland waters whether existing or new are controlled in terms of flow and composition by the Rivers (Prevention of Pollution) Acts 1951 and 1961 (in Scotland, the Rivers (Prevention of Pollution) (Scotland) Acts 1951 and 1965); discharges via wells, boreholes or pipes to underground strata in England and Wales are covered by the Water Resources Act 1963;

(ii) new discharges to estuaries in England and Wales are similarly controlled by the Clean Rivers (Estuaries and Tidal Waters) Act 1960;

(iii) existing discharges to estuarine waters can be controlled by a Tidal Waters order if the regional water authority applies for power to do so; however, few estuaries are in fact controlled by this means;

(iv) new and existing discharges to estuarine waters in Scotland are controlled by the river purification authority if the waters are statutorily 'controlled waters' (e.g. the Firth of Forth and the Firth of Clyde) or are made controlled waters by tidal waters orders. All major estuarine waters in Scotland are now controlled;

(v) discharges to sewers in England and Wales are subject to control by the Public Health (Drainage of Trade Premises) Act 1937 and the Public Health Act 1961 (Part V), and in Scotland by the Sewerage (Scotland) Act 1968.

115. Implementation of Part II of the Control of Pollution Act 1974, dealing

with pollution of water, would impose substantial capital expenditure on water authorities at a time when they are operating under severe capital investment restrictions and when they are under great public pressure to keep their charges as low as possible. In these circumstances, the Government has announced that whilst it would not be reasonable to implement the major provisions of Part II of the Act at the present time, the position is being kept under review. Moreover, it attaches great importance to making the administration of pollution control as open as possible.

116. Responsibility for controlling ingress of mercury to waters and sewage works is vested in the individual regional water authorities in England and Wales and in the drainage authorities (regional and islands councils) in Scotland. More attention is now being paid to routine monitoring of this metal, and as reported previously (HMSO, 1974a), a harmonised water quality monitoring survey has been set up to sample all major rivers just above their tidal limits and at the confluence of principal tributaries. This work includes mercury among the pollutants measured. In addition to water sampling, future work will also involve monitoring biological species; thus fish may be taken and analysed for both total and methylmercury. The regional water authorities and Scottish regional councils and island councils are also responsible for the provision of wholesome drinking water (para. 100) and will now more frequently include mercury in their routine drinking water monitoring programmes, particularly in those cases where either natural levels are higher than usual or where waters are possibly subject to ingress of mercury-containing effluents.

117. The 'Oslo Convention' (Convention for the Prevention of Marine Pollution by Dumping from Ships and Aircraft, Cmnd 4984, HMSO, 1972) and the 'London Convention' (Convention on the Prevention of Marine Pollution by Dumping of Wastes and Other Matter, Cmnd 5169, HMSO, 1972) prohibit the dumping at sea of mercury and its compounds except where these occur as trace contaminants, e.g. in sewage sludges and dredge spoils. The Dumping at Sea Act 1974 implements these Conventions and prohibits the dumping of all substances and materials at sea, except in accordance with a licence granted by the appropriate licensing authority. These are in England and Wales the Ministry of Agriculture, Fisheries and Food, in Scotland the Department of Agriculture and Fisheries for Scotland and in Northern Ireland the Department of the Environment for Northern Ireland.

118. Mercury and its compounds may also reach the seas by discharge from rivers or pipelines which reach the coast. The Control of Pollution Act 1974 enables the UK to ratify the 'Paris Convention' (Convention for the Prevention of Marine Pollution from Land-based Sources, Cmnd 5803, HMSO, 1975). Participating nations undertake in Article 4 to eliminate pollution of the North Sea and North East Atlantic by certain substances, if necessary taking action by stages. The specified substances include mercury and its compounds. Although the Convention is not yet in force, the signatory states have selected mercury for particular attention and a questionnaire has been circulated seeking information on the quantities and concentrations of mercury reaching the sea

from land-based sources in each country. In addition to this Convention, member states of the EEC have recently agreed a Directive on Pollution by Dangerous Substances discharged into the Aquatic Environment (Official Journal No. L129, 18 May 1976). Under this Directive, member states are required to eliminate pollution by mercury and its compounds in inland surface waters, territorial waters, internal coastal waters and ground waters.

Waste disposal

119. Since 1972 the deposit of mercury-bearing wastes has been subject to the provisions of the Deposit of Poisonous Wastes Act. Part I of the Control of Pollution Act 1974 places a responsibility on local authorities to draw up plans for waste disposal and to ensure that adequate facilities for the disposal of all wastes are available. The Government has already announced that whilst it will not be possible in the near future to make resources available to carry out the surveys and plans provided for by Section 2 of the Act, Sections 3 to 11, which provide for a disposal licensing system, command a higher priority. Funds have been transferred to enable local authorities to operate the new system, which was brought into effect in England and Wales on 14 June 1976. The programme of bringing provisions of the Act into force in Scotland is being separately considered. The Department of the Environment some time ago established a number of expert Working Groups to study and advise on problems arising in disposal of specially hazardous materials; one of these groups is currently considering mercury-contaminated materials. The Group's recommendations will form the basis for a Technical Memorandum, incorporating a Code of Practice, which will deal with sources of wastes and handling and disposal requirements. The Group's views will also be taken into account in deciding what controls should be imposed on mercury containing wastes under Section 17 of the Control of Pollution Act in addition to those applied by the licensing system. Other Working Groups are studying the disposal of sewage sludge to land, to the seas and by incineration and here, too, mercury is being considered.

Monitoring and research

120. As mentioned in paragraph 41, the Ministry of Agriculture, Fisheries and Food set up the Working Party on the Monitoring of Foodstuffs for Heavy Metals following reports of high levels of mercury in canned tuna in the USA. The Working Party's objectives are, inter alia, to determine the amounts of mercury (and other heavy metals) in food in the UK and to make reports. The Working Party operates a continuous monitoring programme for the presence of mercury and other heavy metals in the national diet through the Total Diet Study and the analysis of individual food items. It submits its findings to the Food Additives and Contaminants Committee who, after consulting the Toxicity Sub-Committee, advise Ministers what action, if any, is needed. The two reports issued to date on mercury (HMSO, 1971, 1973a) were reassuring but the situation is being kept under review.

121. Following an earlier report in this series (HMSO, 1974a), a set of

Monitoring Management Groups has been set up to consider the monitoring needs of the various sectors of the environment (air, fresh water, the marine environment and land) and the needs in terms of biological and human health. Under the guidance of the appropriate group, action is being taken to improve monitoring in each of the above sectors, and the particular action taken in the case of mercury has been outlined above at paragraphs 113 (air) and 116 (fresh water). The Marine Pollution Monitoring Management Group co-ordinates monitoring of the marine environment and mercury is one of the substances measured in its monitoring programme. The Land Pollution Group will review existing monitoring arrangements for assessment of pollution problems concerning land use practices including disposal of wastes. The groups concerned with biological and human health will co-ordinate and integrate the monitoring activities undertaken by the various groups and provide assessments of the results of monitoring in terms of the likely human or biological hazard.

122. A great deal of research on mercury as a pollutant has recently been and is currently being sponsored by the Government and Research Councils. This work covers mercury in the atmosphere, freshwaters, estuaries, coastal and oceanic waters and their sediments, soils, plants and food, and animals.

123. The recent work on atmospheric mercury includes monitoring of air at a number of rural sites; monitoring of air and rain at other sites of industrial significance and the effect of mercury on human and animal health and on vegetation; a survey of relative atmospheric burdens of mercury in a number of areas by collection and analysis of mosses; and methods for studying the importance of atmospheric deposition of mercury to the marine environment.

124. Much emphasis is given to projects relating to mercury in the aquatic environment. Here, studies have been made of the sources of mercury in the sea (including wind-borne dust and sea water detritus); the nature, concentration, reaction and analysis of inorganic and organic forms of mercury in fresh and marine waters; the background concentrations of mercury in waters and organisms; the distribution of mercury in the water, sediments and biota of e.g. mountain streams, rivers and sea water, with particular reference to local sources of pollution; the mercury contents of suspended solids and sediments of British lakes; the flux of mercury through estuaries and the influence of salinity and temperature on chemical forms of mercury and on mercury uptake by organisms; the mercury contents of sediments from the Mersey, Thames, Forth and Clyde estuaries; the association of inorganic and organic mercurials with individual minerals in sediments from the Severn estuary; a mercury inventory of the Wyre estuary and the residence time in sediments contaminated by industrial mercury-containing effluents; the mercury content of materials forming the ocean floor and the effect of dumping sewage sludge at sea; reactions at the water-marine sediment interface, including the role played by organisms; and processes maintaining the geochemical balance of the seas.

125. Aquatic life has also been studied in detail. This work includes the effect of mercury on marine phytoplankton and zooplankton, their capacity for and

the mechanisms by which they concentrate mercury; the influence of mercury on the growth and distribution of seaweeds around the coasts; the physiology of mercury tolerance by algae in relation to known sources of pollution; the usefulness of seaweeds as indicators of pollution; the effect of mercury on growth of sand-living ciliates; the uptake and excretion of mercury and methylmercury by fish and shell-fish, using both stable and radioactively-labelled mercury; uptake and excretion by fish in coastal and estuarial areas known to be mercury-rich; mechanisms of accumulation and biochemical and behavioural effects of sub-lethal amounts of mercury on organisms; the influence of sub-lethal mercury on physiology and mortality of fish and crustacea from areas naturally and industrially rich in mercury; total mercury and methylmercury levels in fish as biological indication of river water quality; the use of sessile (non-mobile) invertebrates as pollution indicators; and the accumulation of sub-lethal mercury, and associated biochemical effects, through food chains over long periods of time.

126. With regard to the terrestrial pathways of mercury to man, recent and current work covers sampling and analysis of soils and plants, mercury levels in peat, garden soils, arable and non-agricultural soils and the influence of mercurial seed treatments; mercury soil content as a function of depth; sources of mercury in soils in urban areas, in areas where base metal mining has been carried out and around sulphide ore bodies; mercury content of sewage sludges; uptake, transport and accumulation of mercury by a variety of plants (e.g. herbage, grasses, vegetables, perennials) grown under widely-differing conditions, e.g. on normal field and garden soils, on soils treated with mercury salts or sewage sludges or contaminated with industrial chloralkali wastes; and the mercury content of foods in the UK, with special attention being paid to fish, particularly those coming from waters known or suspected to be mercury rich.

127. Wild life is also currently being studied. A reconnaisance survey of heavy metals, including mercury, in British birds has been in progress for about three years and livers from about 70 species from different geographical areas have been analysed. This work includes mercury in the livers and eggs of species of fish-eating seabirds (e.g. guillemots, gannets, puffins and kittiwakes) and its relationship with the distribution of mercury in British waters; mercury in estuarine species such as the Knot, Dunlin, Redshank and Snipe; in wildfowl such as the Mallard, Teal and Widgeon; mercury in owls; and mercury in individual birds exposed to mercury from seed treatments, either directly as in the case of seed-eating farmland birds or indirectly as in the case of predators like the Kestrel.

128. Some research has also been carried out on small mammals such as the field mouse and bank vole living in and around wheat fields where mercury treated seeds are used and on large mammals such as the otter and badger.

129. More detail about the research projects outlined here is given in the "Index of Current Government and Government-supported Research in Environmental Pollution in Great Britain, 1974", available from the Department

of the Environment* and also in "Pollution Research and the Research Councils; Revised List of Projects, 1973" and "1975" (in press) and " Research Grants to the Natural Environmental Sciences", Publication Series D, No. 4, 1973, which are available from the Natural Environment Research Council.†
The Department of the Environment has set up a register of UK research projects (recently completed and in progress) on subjects relating to the Department's interests, including environmental pollution. There is a free enquiry service giving access to the information and this is available to research workers, institutions, organisations commissioning and planning research and the professions. Part IV of the Register of Research, on environmental pollution, became available in 1975. More details of the scheme were given in DOE Press Notice 795, 25 October 1974 (see Appendix III).

130. It is clear from the outline of research given above that there has been extensive coverage of many components of our environment. One purpose of this research is to improve our knowledge of the ways in which mercury is transported through the environment and ultimately to man. However, apart from studies of people occupationally exposed, there has been little research on people exposed to higher than average levels of mercury intake from the general environment. Some more research is being initiated on the heavy metal (including mercury) intakes of special groups of people, e.g. living in special areas or eating particular foods or foods grown on particular soils, and the effect of such exposures upon the health of these people will where necessary be studied by clinical and biological examinations.

---

*Headquarters Library (Research Section)
 Department of the Environment
 2 Marsham Street
 London SW1P 3EB

†Natural Environment Research Council
 Alhambra House
 27-33 Charing Cross Road
 London WC2H 0AX

CHAPTER 5

CONCLUSIONS

131. It is clear that the average person in the UK is at no discernible risk from exposure to mercury. The average intake from food, the major source, is far below the proposed provisional tolerable limit and the possibility of significant exposure from sources such as air, pesticides or pharmaceuticals is very limited. The possibility of excessive occupational exposure is restricted by careful control of environmental concentrations at the work place and, in some cases, by medical screening. Similarly, the environment itself is, as a whole, not being subjected to detrimental effects by emissions of mercury, although locally high concentrations do exist in certain areas and sectors. In spite of this reassuring picture, it is necessary, in order to ensure the continued safety of our environment and of human health, to develop a comprehensive knowledge of the concentration and distribution of mercury (and other pollutants) in all parts of the environment, and a detailed understanding of the pathways by which mercury is transported through the environment and of the effects of mercury on living things. An adequate system of control of emissions, on the lines of the principles outlined in paragraph 95, is also essential.

Monitoring and surveillance

132. An integrated monitoring system for the UK has been described previously (HMSO, 1974a). However, because resources are limited and because in general, exposure to mercury is low, the best use of available resources will be made by examining, at this stage, those situations where exposure is known or expected to be higher than average. There is a dearth of information on the concentrations of both volatile and particulate mercury occurring in air in a number of situations. In particular, we are not certain of the typical levels of mercury vapour present in rural and urban areas, or of levels of particulates in urban areas. We know very little about atmospheric mercury inside the home and information is required about the influences of e.g. the chloralkali industry, coal-burning and metal-processing on local atmospheric concentrations. The sampling requirements demanded by mercury's volatility render it unsuitable for inclusion in the national network of 20 sites currently being set up to monitor airborne particulates and individual monitoring schemes are therefore being initiated; these will concentrate, in the first instance, on monitoring in areas where concentrations are likely to be higher than average.

133. Monitoring of freshwaters has already started under the harmonized monitoring scheme previously announced (HMSO, 1974a). All major rivers are being sampled just above tidal limits and at the confluence of principal tributaries

and data on mercury are already becoming available. There is a need to obtain information on mercury levels in drinking water, and this may become important in relation to an EEC initiative on limits for the metallic content of drinking water.

134. Further research is desirable on the conversion of mercury to the various forms in the environment, particularly to and from methylmercury compounds, and on pathways of mercury through the environment, especially across the water/sediment interface in the freshwater, estuarine and marine environments.

135. Mercury on land is important in relation to the disposal of mercury-containing wastes by landfill and to the practice of using sewage sludges as manures. The Working Group on Disposal of Mercury-containing Wastes, set up by the Department of the Environment, is examining the first of these and a Code of Practice stressing the importance of monitoring will be published. Other Working Groups are examining the disposal of sewage sludge to land, to the seas and by incineration and they too will be providing Codes of Practice, identifying acceptable conditions for each of these categories of use or disposal.

136. Biological surveillance and monitoring are as important as monitoring the physical environment directly because in this way only can the amounts of mercury available to living things, particularly those which form part of man's diet, be determined. Most attention has been given to the aquatic environment and results have proved reassuring. However, levels of mercury in fish from certain areas are higher than usual and these will continue to be monitored as described in paragraph 120. The control of dumping now being exercised through the Dumping at Sea Act 1974 will ensure that unacceptable amounts of mercury do not reach the sea in this way, but there is a need also to continue to control discharges from rivers and pipelines and this is clearly a question of control at the stage of effluent generation. Birds are also being monitored for mercury residues but the experience gained in Scotland has shown that higher residues are only likely to occur in some wild and game birds at times of sowing of cereal seeds treated with mercury.

137. Monitoring of human health is important for those occupationally exposed to mercury and this is the responsibility of the Health and Safety Executive. There are several groups of people who are exposed to mercury but who are not examined at present; these include people working in and handling mercury in dental practices. It is evident that excessive absorption has occurred in the past, probably largely through respiration of high concentrations of mercury resulting from poor handling techniques; it is important that atmospheric concentrations of mercury in the dental surgery should be maintained below the threshold limit value recommended by the Health and Safety Executive, and advice has been provided on this by the British Dental Association. Those working in dental practices should be regularly examined for excessive mercury absorption and this may need to be extended to the families of dentists where the surgery itself forms part of the dentist's home and where members of the families may be exposed.

138. It would also be of interest to study exposure to mercury in the families of those working in the mercury-using industries, of families living near major sources of atmospheric mercury and of any people who can be found to have a higher than usual intake of mercury from food. If higher than average exposure were found in the first group, there would be a need to know how the mercury was transported from the work place to the home and whether the excessive exposure would be likely to affect the children. It would be necessary to include exposure to elemental, inorganic and organic forms of mercury by choice of suitable industries. It should be noted, however, that great care is usually exercised in mercury-using industries to preclude the possibility of transport of mercury to the home; this includes provision of showering and washing facilities and changes of clothing.

139. The mercury levels in people eating greater than usual quantities of fish with a high mercury content have already been examined (HMSO, 1971). The results proved reassuring but there was great difficulty in identifying such people and in the event the number examined was only six. There is a need for more work on unusual dietary exposure. Moreover, fish with a high mercury content may find their way predominantly to particular local market outlets; if so, this would amplify their importance. The consumption of wild birds, such as wood pigeons, which have fed on mercury-treated seeds has also been mentioned. Whilst people eating large amounts of pigeon meat might be an example of a specially-exposed group meriting study (if such a group could be identified), the first priority in the use of scarce resources should be given to keeping a watching brief on mercury levels in the pigeons themselves.

140. The work carried out by MAFF on the monitoring of food for mercury has been reassuring, even where unusual dietary habits have been encountered but the number of such people examined has been very small. Whilst the majority of the population eat a diet near to 'average', there is a possibility that there are small numbers of people who eat diets very different from the average. Future work should pay attention to establishing dietary intakes of mercury and other toxic metals by such people. Preliminary steps have already been taken by MAFF in this direction, but as experienced previously, such people are difficult to identify.

Toxicology

141. Many different forms of mercury are currently in use and there are a number of ways in which mercury can reach living things and a variety of chemical changes possible along some routes through the environment. The number of different living things exposed to mercury is large and each may have an individual reaction to mercury of any type. For these reasons, a comprehensive and detailed knowledge of the toxicology of mercury would require considerable resources. The greatest priority has been given to understanding the toxicity of mercury compounds to man and while the details of toxicological investigations have not been discussed in this Report, it is evident that further research is needed; first, on the mechanisms of toxic action of mercury and,

secondly, on low level exposure (in particular to organic compounds) over long periods of time.

Control of use and emissions

142. Although the conclusions emerging about average exposure to mercury in the UK are reassuring, mercury is a toxic substance with no known biological function. It is therefore desirable on health grounds that man's exposure to mercury be kept as low as practicable. There is clearly no need for precipitate action which would result in significant and unnecessary economic and social costs. However, where excessive contamination of the environment exists, or is likely to arise, steps should be taken as and when appropriate progressively to reduce man-made contributions, taking into account not only the desirability of improving safety margins still further but also industrial economic viability, technical adequacy and the availability of less hazardous alternatives. Where a pathway by which mercury might reach man is known, special care is needed; this may involve more stringent control over releases of mercury to the environment.

143. The chloralkali industry is one of the major sources of emissions, but this industry is vital both to other industries and because much of the chlorine produced is essential for the maintenance of wholesome water supplies. Much progress has been made in recent years in developing treatment processes for reducing losses of mercury to air and the industry has already planned extensions of the use of such processes: further extensions may yet be necessary. Reductions have also been made in emissions to water and both new and established plant is being equipped with improved treatment processes; this is particularly important wherever such mercury may find its way, directly or indirectly, to man. Furthermore, one major chlorine-producing company has indicated to Government that it plans to use the alternative diaphragm process, which uses no mercury, in any additional future production plant in the UK, beyond that already planned and under construction. There has been a considerable swing towards the use of this type of plant abroad, and in Japan all chloralkali plant will have to use this method by 1978.

144. The use of mercury compounds in paints is one aspect of the non-agricultural use of pesticides. As a consequence of an earlier report in this series, Pollution Paper No. 3, "The Non-Agricultural Uses of Pesticides in Great Britain" (HMSO, 1974b), the Government and the paint industry are jointly reviewing the need to continue the use of mercury compounds in paints.

145. The disposal of mercury-containing wastes has been mentioned above at paragraph 135. This is a significant aspect of the control of emissions, accounting for upwards of 100 tonnes of mercury annually, including that contained in primary batteries and industrial and sewage sludges.

146. Agricultural and related uses of mercury compounds, particularly as seed treatments, play an important part in maintaining the level of our domestic food production and their value must be recognised. Alternative pesticides are

now appearing but none has yet been shown to be as effective under UK conditions as mercury for treating seeds for all major cereals and sugar beet and only one has so far been approved for efficacy as a cereal seed treatment under the Agricultural Chemicals Approval Scheme, and then solely for use on winter wheat. Research is continuing in this field. An Expert Group convened by the Food and Agriculture Organisation and the World Health Organisation has recommended (WHO, 1974) that (i) the use of alkylmercury compounds as seed treatments should be strictly limited to the treatment of nuclear stocks of cereal seed used for the first few generations of seed multiplication. They should never be permitted for the treatment of cereal seed to be exported for the production of food; and (ii) alkoxyalkylmercury and arylmercury compounds should be used to treat cereal seed only if the need for such treatment has been evaluated and the possible use of an alternative ruled out. They should be permitted for use on cereal seed to be exported for the production of food only if safeguards exist to prevent the possibility of the seed being diverted from its intended use. As safeguards, detailed recommendations are made on dyeing of grain to indicate the presence of mercurial pesticides, on labelling, packaging, handling and associated documentation (in the appropriate language or dialect). The Advisory Committee on Pesticides and Other Toxic Chemicals has in hand a detailed review of the use of mercury in agricultural pesticides and in that review will take into account the recommendations of the expert group convened by FAO/WHO.

APPENDIX I

SOURCES AND CONCENTRATIONS OF MERCURY

D

APPENDIX I

SOURCES AND CONCENTRATIONS OF MERCURY

The natural mercury cycle

A.1. Mercury or mercury compounds occur naturally in trace quantities in all parts of the environment. Some details are given in Tables 1–3 and discussed later.

A.2. Degassing of crustal materials and terrestrial volcanic activity (Eshleman et al, 1971; Siegel et al, 1973) release mercury to the atmosphere in elemental and particulate form, i.e. as vapour and as finely-divided solid mercury compounds. Up to about 150,000 tonnes of mercury are possibly mobilised each year in this way (Weiss et al, 1971). Earth's molten core also enriches igneous rocks with mercury and creates new mercury-bearing rocks where tectonic plates are moving apart, e.g. along the mid-Atlantic ridge. (The results of this movement are sometimes seen in spectacular fashion when new islands such as Surtsey emerge.)

A.3. Natural erosion of rocks and mineral deposits by weathering transport mercury into the hydrosphere (rivers, lakes and seas) at a rate variously estimated from 230–5,000 tonnes annually (Table 2). Submarine leaching, erosion and volcanic activity must also transport mercury from sub-marine rocks and sediments and from Earth's core to the seas, but the total quantity involved does not appear to have been estimated. Certainly, however, anomalously high mercury concentrations have been found in waters near the mid-Atlantic ridge (Carr et al, 1974; Olafsson, 1975). In view of the fact that water covers the major part of Earth's surface and that many tectonic junctions are known to occur under the sea, it seems likely that substantial quantities of mercury are naturally released to oceans by sub-marine activities.

A.4. Movement of mercury from the atmosphere to marine and freshwaters occurs in rain and dustfall and these together possibly amount to about 50,000 tonnes of mercury per year (Peakall and Lovett, 1972). The reverse movement occurs by evaporation, but to a much smaller extent, possibly about 2,000 tonnes/annum (Peakall and Lovett, 1972).

A.5. Mercury in waters is often preferentially adsorbed on to sediments and suspended particulates; some reverse movement by oxidative extraction or absorption may also occur. Uptake of mercury from waters and sediments by aquatic organisms may be accompanied by considerable concentration; decay and leaching form the reverse path. Mercury may also be transported into the biosphere (living plant and animal tissue) via uptake from soils; excretion, death and decay reverse the process. Direct transfer of mercury from the atmosphere to the biosphere occurs in uptake by mosses and other plants; here decay and evaporation form the reverse path, but much of this mercury will be deposited in soils when the moss dies.

A.6. Movement of mercury from sediments to igneous rocks occurs by metamorphosis over geological time periods, and from sediments to Earth's core in regions where destruction of crustal material is taking place, i.e. where tectonic plates are moving together, e.g. off Japan.

A.7. We know little of the relative magnitudes of this complex system of mercury mobilisation. However, calculations made so far suggest that degassing and volcanic activity are by far the most important mechanism by which mercury is naturally mobilised.

Man's use of mercury

A.8. Mercury ores occur in exploitable quantities in Spain, the USSR, Italy, the USA, Mexico, Canada, Yugoslavia, China, Japan, Turkey, Ireland and the Philippines; they do not exist in the UK. The first seven of these countries are the major producers. Total known reserves of mercury, exploitable at current prices, exceed 200,000 tonnes, almost half of which occur in Spain (Brobst and Pratt, 1973). World mercury consumption has fallen slightly in recent years to about 9,000 tonnes, due to environmental pressures on a number of uses. The UK's requirement is met largely by imports, of which Spain and the EEC supply about 30 per cent. *Net* imports (i.e. imports less exports) in recent years have varied from 235–788 tonnes. UK production of mercury, amounting to something of the order of 100 tonnes/year, is confined to refining of used mercury by e.g. acid treatment and redistillation.

A.9. In addition to the metal, small amounts of mercuric oxide ($25 \cdot 5$ tonnes in 1973) and mercuric sulphide ($0 \cdot 3$ tonne in 1973) are also imported into the UK. Although we import all our simple alkylmercury compounds, the UK is a net exporter of organomercury products generally, the quantities ranging from 125–500 tonnes annually over the period 1970–1973. (The quantity of mercury expressed as metal in these compounds would be ca 47–57 tonnes per year).

A.10. The principle uses of mercury and its compounds in the UK occur in:
(i) the chemical industry – production of chlorine and caustic soda (in 1975, total mercury supplied, 475 tonnes, of which 283 tonnes were used); in household paints (30 tonnes) and in marine anti-fouling paints (up to 4 tonnes); as a catalyst in polymer and dyestuffs production (up to about 11 tonnes); in laboratory chemicals (10 tonnes);
(ii) the electrical industry – in primary batteries including mercury cells and other types (80 tonnes); fluorescent lamps, electrical, measuring and control equipment (including thermometers, barometers and polarographs) (14 tonnes);
(iii) agriculture and related uses – inorganic and organic compounds used as fungicides, insecticides and herbicides (a total of about 28 tonnes);
(iv) dentistry – in the preparation of mercury amalgam fillings (30 tonnes).

43

Minor uses occur in the pharmaceutical and medical industry (as antiseptic preservatives to protect creams) and also in special soaps and ammoniated bleach creams produced for export (about 2 tonnes); in adhesives, principally for ceramic tiles (about 1 tonne); and in munitions, pigments, photography, fireworks, laboratory vacuum pumps, textile fungicides etc. (totalling about 6 tonnes). Mercury compounds were previously used as slimicides in pulp and paper mills and in cooling towers. Each of these uses can, in one way or another, result in release of mercury to some part of the environment. In addition to these sources, mercury is released during the combustion of coal, oil and natural gas, in production of cement, in the disposal of mercury-containing wastes, and from metallurgical processes.

The chloralkali process

A.11. The major use of mercury in the UK, and indeed in the world, occurs in the simultaneous production of chlorine and caustic soda by electrolysis of sodium chloride solution (brine). Two different types of electrolytic cell are in use today, the mercury cell and the diaphragm cell; only the former is of relevance to this report. About 90 per cent of UK chlorine/caustic soda production utilises this type of cell, because it is more flexible in operation than the diaphragm cell and because the overall energy costs (taking into account costs associated with the purification of the caustic soda necessary with the diaphragm cell) are about 10 per cent lower.

A.12. The mercury cell consists basically of a container holding brine, in which is a graphite anode (more recently coated titanium) and through which flows a mercury stream acting as a cathode. Electrolysis liberates chlorine gas at the anode and sodium at the cathode. The sodium forms an amalgam with the flowing mercury and is continuously removed from the cell thereby. Water is then added to the amalgam, releasing caustic soda and hydrogen gas, together with mercury which is re-cycled to the cell. The possible sources of mercury release to the external environment are:

(i) as a vapour in the hydrogen gas or hydrogen vents;
(ii) in ventilation of the cell room, the atmosphere of which contains mercury vapour;
(iii) as a trace impurity in the caustic soda, which is used extensively in the manufacture of cosmetics, detergents, soaps, pulp and paper and textiles;
(iv) in waste brine and wash-waters from the cell room;
(v) in spent brine sludges and contaminated solids which are deposited in controlled areas, e.g. embanked areas of salt marsh land.

Mercury is also lost to structures (e.g. walls and floors) wherever it is used.

A.13. Until recent years, losses of mercury from chloralkali plants probably totalled about 250 g per tonne of chlorine produced. Today, after considerable expenditure by industry, losses of mercury for each tonne of chlorine produced probably average about 22 g to air (items (i) and (ii) above), 18 g to water (item (iv)) and about 1·4 g in products (item (iii)). The hydrogen stream contains,

44

after cooling, about 3·6 g of mercury per tonne of chlorine produced. Special treatment methods, such as molecular sieves or iodised charcoal filters, designed to produce very low residual mercury concentrations, are used where the hydrogen is sent for special application, but surplus hydrogen is usually burnt without such special treatment. Purging and venting of 'weak' hydrogen from the caustic soda leaving the 'end-boxes' of the cells is the largest single source of mercury loss to the atmosphere within this process, accounting for 10–25 g/tonne chlorine. Treatment processes for this weak hydrogen have only recently been developed; one is operating in the UK and another is planned. Ventilation of the cell room may account for a loss of 1·5–7·5 g of mercury per tonne of chlorine, but modern cell rooms, with atmospheric concentrations of about 15 $\mu g/m^3$ (well below the threshold limit value, published by HM Factory Inspectorate, of 50 $\mu g/m^3$) will typically lose about 1·5–2·5 g of mercury/tonne chlorine. Finally, mercury recovery on site by pyrolysis and distillation of various process residues produces a minor loss to air of about 0·2–0·6 g/tonne chlorine.

A.14. There are nine chloralkali plants in the UK, eight of which use mercury cells, and the total chlorine production capacity is about 1 million tonnes. The overall use of mercury by the chloralkali industry in 1975 amounted to 283 tonnes, with 193 tonnes being put to stock. Total emissions were about 18 tonnes to aqueous effluents, 18 tonnes to air by ventilation, 4 tonnes to hydrogen gas and 1·4 tonnes to the alkali: 167 tonnes of the total use by the chloralkali industry were unaccounted for by measurements.

A.15. In addition to the above, mercury finds its way into the waste solids (brine sludges containing up to about 600 ppm mercury) which are deposited in embanked areas of salt marsh land. This mercury cannot be regarded as freely mobilised: mercury levels in run-off waters are low and there is no evidence of any biological methylation occurring. Nevertheless, this represents an accumulation of some 73 tonnes of mercury for 1975.

Paints

A.16. The use of mercury compounds in paints has recently been reviewed (HMSO, 1974b). The largest proportion of the total use occurs in general decorative paints (mainly emulsion paints), in which the mercury compounds (usually phenylmercury compounds) are incorporated as general biocides at concentrations of about 0·001–0·05 per cent, expressed as mercury by weight. Much if not all of this mercury, which comprises 30 tonnes annually, must eventually be released to the environment. Mercury compounds (usually phenylmercury dimethyldithiocarbamate or chloride) are also used as anti-fouling formulations in marine paints, but here the mercury concentration is much higher, 2–5 per cent by weight. The efficacy of these paints depends upon the slow release of the toxin and a proportion of these substances therefore end up in the sea. Here the quantity used in the UK amounts to 4 tonnes of mercury per year. The use of mercury compounds in adhesives, e.g. wallpaper pastes, has declined in recent years and is now very small (HMSO, 1974b).

Catalysis

A.17. Mercury catalysts are used in the manufacture of elastomeric poly-urethanes and here traces of the catalyst end up in the product. The estimated annual consumption of mercury in the UK in this application is 2 tonnes. Most of this will ultimately be disposed of by landfill. The dyestuffs industry also uses mercuric sulphate catalysts in the manufacture of anthraquinone sulphonic acid dyestuffs, some 5–10 tonnes of mercury equivalent as oxide being used annually in the UK. Some of the mercury goes into the product and the rest into waste sludges. Mercury catalysts are no longer used in the UK in the production of vinyl chloride and vinyl acetate.

The electrical industry

A.18. Mercury is used in fluorescent and mercury discharge lamps, power rectifiers, switches and primary batteries, including mercury cells, alkali-manganese, silver-zinc and zinc-carbon types. There are about 30 mg of mercury in each fluorescent tube, which on the estimated number of 100 million installed lamps in the UK, gives some 3 tonne of mercury contained in such fittings. A replacement rate of 10 per cent per annum would mean that about 0·3 tonne would probably be deposited in landfill sites each year. Recovery of mercury from mercury-containing power rectifiers is common although some disposal to tips may occur, but these rectifiers are being replaced by more efficient solid-state devices. Mercury switches are also being superseded by solid-state devices in some applications. The greatest use of mercury in this category occurs in the production of primary batteries, now widely used in domestic, industrial, office and medical equipment. This use accounted for a total of 80 tonnes of mercury in 1975, and 47 tonnes in such goods for export. About 1 million batteries, equivalent to less than 1 tonne of mercury, are imported annually. Some recovery of these items is taking place but an unknown though substantial quantity of mercury must be finding its way into rubbish tips as batteries and equipment are discarded. Electrical apparatus and control instruments accounted for 14 tonnes of mercury in 1975.

Agriculture

A.19. Both inorganic and organic forms of mercury are used in agriculture and related areas in the UK. Inorganic compounds, mainly mercurous and mercuric chloride, are used to control diseases of brassica crops, onion seed and sports turf; in gardens, some of these compounds are used for elimination of moss from lawns. The total quantity used is about 15 tonnes annually (expressed as the metal), and the total area treated about 8,000 hectares (ha). Dosages range from about 0·50 kg/ha for the lowest application rate on brassicae to about 13 kg/ha for the heaviest of the onion treatments.

A.20. Organic compounds are used on about 3·2 million hectares annually in the UK. The most widespread use is as cereal seed treatment, where the rate of application (expressed as the metal) averages 4 g/ha over about 3 million hectares. The most commonly used compounds here are phenylmercury acetate and ethylmercury chloride but small quantities of phenylmercury urea (ca 10 per cent of treatments) are also used. The total quantity of mercury used here is about 12 tonnes annually. The next most widespread use is on sugar beet seed over some 180,000 ha at a dosage of less than 3 g/ha; here ethylmercury phosphate is used. In addition, methoxylethylmercury acetate (or chloride) is used for seed potato and bulb dips. The total quantity of mercury used for beet seed, seed potatoes and bulb dips is about 0·5 tonne/year. About 20,000 ha of fruit trees are treated at a mean dosage of ca 45 g/ha and there is a little use (ca 1,000 ha) to control turf diseases; in both of these applications phenylmercury acetate predominates, the total usage being about 1 tonne/year.

A.21. Overall, therefore, the use of mercury compounds in agriculture and related uses amounts to about 28 tonnes annually or about 5 per cent of the UK annual consumption; only about 1·2 tonnes of this is in the form of alkylmercury compounds. All of these compounds have been cleared under the Pesticides Safety Precautions Scheme (paragraph 107, Chapter 4) and safe uses have been agreed with the Government Departments concerned.

A.22. Mercury compounds may be applied as powders adhering to pre-treated seeds; as liquids absorbed onto seed coats, the skin of seed potatoes or bulb scales; as liquids applied directly as sprays to fruit and other crops and as dusts applied either in slurry form direct to the roots of transplants or to the soil itself. Mercury may also occur in sewage sludges used as crop manures.

A.23. Mercury compounds may be absorbed on the humus fraction of soil, particularly under acid conditions, and on the mineral colloids in less-acid conditions (Andersson, 1967). Leaching of mercury can occur from certain soils, particularly sands (MacLean et al, 1975), but leaching hardly occurs from clays, sandy clays or peats (Poelstra et al, 1973).

A.24. The high volatility of some of the organic mercurial fungicides and breakdown resulting in the formation of mercury vapour leads to some loss to the atmosphere during treatment and storage of seeds and during field application (Lord et al, 1971). When they reach the soil, mercury compounds behave in different ways, depending, inter alia, on the chemical, physical and biological properties of the compound and of the soil itself, and on the wetness and temperature of the soil. Applications of mercuric chloride, phenyl, ethyl and methylmercury compounds can all be degraded in soil into mercury vapour, which can volatilise into the atmosphere (Zimmerman and Crocker, 1933; Kimura and Miller, 1964; Frear and Dills, 1967). Some organic mercurials are degraded to other more volatile organics, to inorganic forms (Bache et al, 1973) or, by certain organisms, into metallic mercury (Furukawa et al, 1969).

A.25. Methylation of mercury compounds can occur in soil, being activated either by micro-organisms (Beck et al, 1974; Ben-Bassat et al, 1972; Yamada and Tonomura, 1972) or chemically (Kim et al, 1970). High concentrations of mercury inhibit the microbial activity, but at the usual levels of mercury in soil (ca 0·1 ppm) no inhibition is to be expected.

A.26. In summary, the concentrations of the various forms of mercury in the soil are a function of that naturally present, additions from atmospheric fall-out (rain and dust) and agricultural applications, additions from upward movements of geological mercury, losses from volatilisation into the atmosphere following degradation, small losses from leaching and small losses carried off in crop residues.

A.27. The use of organomercury compounds as cereal seed treatments over the past few decades has greatly improved cereal yields. Conditions prevailing in the early part of this century, when bunt or stinking smut of wheat and covered smut and leaf stripe of barley were serious problems, would indicate that about 30–35 per cent of wheat seed might be unsuitable for sowing if treatment were discontinued since the resulting crops would be discounted for milling, and that comparable losses in barley and oats would result (Hewett, 1974; Strickland, 1967). It is also important to recognise that seed-borne diseases have strong powers of recovery from very low levels of incidence and therefore that to stop treatment of seed stocks for more than one year is probably undesirable (Hewett, 1974). Since 1970, several countries have approved legislation which bans or severely restricts the use of mercury in agriculture (although some re-introduction has taken place for special purposes). As a result of restrictions, several non-mercurial seed treatments have emerged. Some are already available commercially and others are still being evaluated. In the UK, three non-mercurial fungicide treatments are available for cereal seed. Similar products are being evaluated in mainland Europe. These products are mixtures of a novel chemical and a traditional fungicide, and fungicide mixtures appear necessary to achieve a wide spectrum of disease control and to make the products more economically attractive. At present, the new treatments are up to 10 times more costly than mercury treatments, largely because of the high dosage rates necessary. Only one has yet been approved for efficacy under UK conditions and then solely for use on winter wheat.

A.28. Organomercury steeps and dips are used for sugar beet seed protection and to treat diseases on seed potatoes and flower bulbs. Alternatives are coming into use for potato treatment, but ethylmercury phosphate remains an important protectant for beet seed. Similarly, the use of organomercurials in controlling apple and pear scab is declining as alternatives come into use but mercury sprays remain particularly useful for cleaning up orchards badly infected.

A.29. The inorganic mercury compounds are mainly used to control Club Root in brassicae and White Rot in onions. Alternatives are costly and more work is needed here. The other substantial use, in controlling moss and fungi in turf, is declining slowly as iron compounds, sometimes with added herbicide, come into use.

A.30. As mentioned earlier, mercury may also occur in sewage sludges, a proportion of which are used as fertilisers. The mercury content of sludges varies widely, but the mean for sludges arising in agricultural areas is about 1–3 ppm (dry solids); higher levels occur, usually in sludges arising in industrial areas. If spread at a realistic rate of 50–65 tonnes of dry solids/ha every five to six years, then the rate in annual terms is not very different from the rate used in top fruit sprays, and is about an order of magnitude lower than dosages for mercury used on sports turf, brassicae and other vegetables. The spreading of sewage sludge may lead to an accumulation of mercury in agricultural or horticultural soils. The advisability of spreading sewage sludge on any particular soil depends upon, amongst other things, the mercury content of the sludge and the soil in question.

A.31. The use of mercury in agriculture has received much attention because here the material is deliberately introduced into the environment. However, what is important in the context of these various uses is whether the particular application results in a significantly enhanced availability of mercury to animals or man. It should also be remembered that this use is under positive PSPS control. The significance of agricultural uses is dealt with in paragraphs A.71 and A.72.

Dentistry

A.32. Mercury amalgams have been used as dental fillings for about 150 years and today about 30 tonnes of mercury are used annually for this purpose. During the preparation of fillings and during the drilling out of old fillings, mercury vapour and particulates are released to air. The possibilities of hazards arising to the patient and to dental staff are considered at paragraphs 82 and 83 of Chapter 3.

Paper and pulp

A.33. The processing of vegetable fibres under moist conditions provides an almost ideal medium for the growth of micro-organisms, unless preventive measures are taken. Mercury compounds, particularly phenylmercury acetate, have been used extensively in the past as slimicides in this industry, but a campaign organised by the British Paper and Board Makers' Association (now the British Paper and Board Industries Federation) has succeeded in eliminating their use in the UK (HMSO, 1974b).

Combustion of coal

A.34. The mercury content of coal is variable. A recent survey (Taylor, to be published) of UK coals found average values ranging from 0·054–0·46 ppm, according to the area from which the coal was mined. A few isolated cases of higher concentrations, in the range 1–2 ppm were also observed, but the overall mean was about 0·18 ppm. Another study (Jones and Nickless, 1973) gave a mean of 0·3 ppm (range 0·02–1·44 ppm) for coals from South Wales and a mean of 0·14 ppm (range 0·07–0·3 ppm) for North Somerset coals.

A.35. Very similar results have been reported in a study of North-American coals carried out at the US National Bureau of Standards (Rook et al, 1972). This indicated a range of mercury levels from about 0·05–0·5 ppm with an average level of 0·1–0·2 ppm. This is in close agreement with earlier American work which reported average concentrations of 0·18 ppm for 55 samples of Illinois coals (Ruch et al, 1971) and about 0·2 ppm for a range of American coals (Schlesinger and Schults, 1971). Very different figures were given in a study of 36 American coals (Joensuu, 1971) where the range was 0·07–33 ppm, with an average of 3·3 ppm (although three-quarters of the samples had concentrations below 0·7 ppm) and in Russian work (quoted in Fleischer, 1970) where the average level was about 1 ppm for coals from the Donbass area.

A.36. When coal is burnt mercury may be liberated as vapour in the flue gases or retained in the ash or soot. Mercury balance studies (Billings and Matson, 1972; Auerbach, 1973; Diehl et al, 1972) carried out in America on large coal-fired furnaces indicate that the majority (up to about 90 per cent) of the mercury content of the coal is usually emitted as vapour from the stack, whilst a minor amount remains in the ashes collected at the furnace bottom and in the particulate matter collected in the electrostatic precipitators. The concentration of mercury in the ashes is usually slightly lower than in the coal used to fire the furnace (Rancitelli, 1971; Auerbach, 1973), and is typically 0·1–0·2 ppm, i.e. comparable with the natural background concentration of mercury in soils and rocks. This material therefore represents no environmental hazard.

A.37. The concentration of mercury in the effluent waters from the coal-furnace was below 0·001 ppm and the transport of mercury from the plant to the environment via water thus appears to be a route of only very minor significance (Billings and Matson, 1972).

A.38. The global discharge of mercury to the atmosphere as a consequence of coal-burning has been estimated at 3,000 tonnes/year (Joensuu, 1971). However, this figure is based on an assumed average mercury concentration of 1 ppm, which is almost certainly much too high. Using the average commonly observed in UK and American work of 0·1–0·3 ppm, and a total world use of coal of 3,000 million tonnes, the total emission of mercury to air from coal-burning may be estimated at about 300–900 tonnes/year.

A.39. In the UK, about 120 million tonnes of coal are burnt each year and hence the total annual emission of mercury to air for the UK is probably about 12–36 tonnes. A little over half of this is emitted at high level from the stacks of power stations and other large coal-burning plants and the remainder from domestic fires. Little is known with certainty of the subsequent dispersal of mercury from the stack plume or from domestic chimneys, or of its possible attachment to aerosol particulates, but it is reasonable to suppose that it becomes very widely dispersed and diluted in the atmosphere. Calculations (Lockeretz, 1974) suggest that most of the emissions from high stacks remain airborne for relatively long distances, typically tens of kilometres, though this is dependent upon the size of the particulates emitted and the prevailing meteorological and topographical conditions.

Combustion of oil and natural gas
A.40. The mercury content of crude oils is usually very low (Jones, 1975).

In a survey covering Alaskan, Middle Eastern, African and Californian crudes, levels of $0 \cdot 01$–$0 \cdot 034$ ppm were found; in another survey covering crudes from Libya, Louisiana, Wyoming and California, levels were generally in the range $0 \cdot 02$–$0 \cdot 1$ ppm, but in one case for an oil from the 'Cymric' field (California), the level was $29 \cdot 7$ ppm. This, however, is completely atypical of oils in general and is a consequence of the fact that oil and mercury deposits were adjacent. A realistic mean concentration for all oils is about $0 \cdot 05$ ppm. This is not inconsistent with the measured mercury contents of some heating oils in the USA, values being in the range $0 \cdot 06$–$0 \cdot 07$ ppm.

A.41. In the absence of evidence to the contrary, it is reasonable to suppose that all of the oil's mercury content is released to air during combustion. The total UK use of fuel oils amounts to about 110 million tonnes per year; assuming a mean mercury concentration of $0 \cdot 05$ ppm this corresponds to an annual release of mercury of about $5 \cdot 5$ tonnes. On a global scale, the total annual emission is probably about 125 tonnes. Combustion of oil is therefore only a minor source of mercury emission to the atmosphere.

A.42. Mercury is also present in minute but measurable quantities in natural gas. At the well-head, gas from the Dutch fields was reported to contain about $0 \cdot 22$ ppm of mercury, but this was reduced during cooling, separation and treatment processes by a factor of about 15: further reductions ensue during delivery, with levels at the point of use being about $0 \cdot 001$–$0 \cdot 006$ ppm. Even smaller quantities at the well-head, about $0 \cdot 012$ ppm, have been detected in gas from the North Sea.

Cement production

A.43. Production of cement has often been cited as a major source of mercury emission to the atmosphere. This has presumably been based on the facts that a very large quantity of cement is produced throughout the world and that the materials from which it is produced have a small but measurable mercury content, and on the assumption that the very high temperature involved in production (ca $1500 \degree C$) will drive off the entire mercury content as mercury vapour. In the absence of data to the contrary (i.e. mercury balance studies on cement works), this assumption must be considered reasonable.

A.44. In the UK about 16 million tonnes of cement are produced each year. This necessitates processing about 18 million tonnes of limestone and 7 million tonnes of clay or shale. Taking the mean mercury concentration in these two materials to be ca $0 \cdot 1$ ppm (see Table 3) and assuming that all of it is emitted to air, an emission of about $2 \cdot 5$ tonnes annually is indicated. This is a small amount compared with other sources. It, too, is likely to become widely dispersed and diluted in the atmosphere although no data for this are available.

A.45. Mercury is present in small quantities in all non-ferrous metal concentrates. Typical values are as follows: in zinc concentrates from 4–190 ppm, but usually below 25 ppm; in lead concentrates from 7–160 ppm, usually below 100 ppm; in oxide concentrates, from less than 1–70 ppm, and in tin/copper

51

ores from Cornwall, a mean of ca 0·05 ppm. In general, ores (other than of mercury itself) do not usually contain more than 10–30 ppm of mercury.

A.46. During metallurgical processing of ores such as smelting, some of the mercury content may be emitted as vapour or as mercury bound to particulates. In the absence of mercury balance studies on smelting furnaces, it is not possible to calculate with any degree of precision the total emissions from this source. However, assuming the worst case, namely that *all* of the mercury is emitted during processing, would mean that the metallurgical processing of non-ferrous ores would result in the release of about 5 tonnes of mercury annually in the UK.

A.47. Production of iron and steel also leads to mercury emissions, since mercury is present as a trace contaminant (a mean level of about 0·04 ppm) in limestone and dolomite and in the various ores (a maximum concentration of <2 ppm). Processing of about 4 million tonnes of limestone and dolomite and 22 million tonnes of ore in sinter plants and blast furnaces would lead to a total emission to air of about 44 tonnes of mercury if all ores contained the highest mercury concentrations seen and if all this were emitted. The actual emission is likely to be much smaller than this.

Disposal of sewage sludge

A.48. Mercury in industrial effluents discharged to watercourses may subsequently become concentrated in sewage sludges, which are disposed of by dumping at sea (20 per cent), landfill and incineration (40 per cent) or use as a manure (40 per cent) (HMSO, 1970). Dumping at sea has been a growing practice and in addition to the three large cities of London, Manchester and Glasgow, at least 19 other authorities now dispose of sewage sludge to sea. At the present time the total quantity of sludge disposed of in this way is about 9 million tonnes per year; nearly 5·5 million tonnes goes to the North Sea, over 2 million tonnes to the Irish Sea and the remainder is divided between the Bristol and English Channels (Portmann, 1974). Mercury concentrations in sewage sludge cover a wide range, with an overall mean of about 0·35 ppm but in certain areas, e.g. London and Manchester, the mean is as high as 1–1·5 ppm (HMSO, 1973). (These concentrations are expressed in terms of wet sludge.) About 10 tonnes of mercury enter the seas around England and Wales each year as a consequence of sludge dumping from ships. Considerably greater quantities enter the sea through coastal discharges by pipelines. Mercury concentrations in fish caught in certain coastal waters, e.g. the Thames Estuary and the Eastern Irish Sea, reflect these practices, although the possibility that mercury is derived from other sources cannot be ignored.

A.49. The remaining sewage sludge is either sent for landfill or burnt (ca 16 million tonnes annually) or used as a manure (ca 16 million tonnes annually). If the mean concentration of mercury in this sludge is ca 0·35 ppm (wet weight), then the *total* quantity of mercury dispersed annually in these ways is about 10 tonnes. Some of the mercury in landfill sites might be expected to be slowly volatilised into the atmosphere or, to a lesser extent, leached out by waters. Sludge incinerators probably release some mercury to air but the extent of this is unknown. The significance of mercury in sludge used as manure is discussed in paragraph A.72.

Other emissions

A.50. Losses of mercury to any part of the environment arising out of its use in medical and pharmaceutical products and from miscellaneous laboratory uses such as occur in barometers, thermometers and vacuum pumps are not reliably calculable. However, as a general rule the entire mercury content of pharmaceuticals is likely to be ultimately released to some part of the environment, whereas the content of only those thermometers which are broken is released.

A.51. It has often been suggested that man's annual contribution to mercury in the environment is approximately equal to that naturally mobilised each year, and therefore that man's activities may be having a considerable influence on mercury levels generally. However, a comparison of global industrial emissions, calculated (Gavis and Ferguson, 1972) to be about 5,000 tonnes annually, with those from natural sources reveals that the former are very much smaller in magnitude. The significance of man's emissions is that they are *localised* and may give rise to high concentrations of mercury in some local part of the environment.

Concentrations in the environment

The atmosphere

A.52. Naturally-occurring concentrations of airborne mercury depend on the geographical location (i.e. whether over sea or land and whether mineral deposits are present); on meteorological factors (wind speed and direction, the presence of fog, the occurrence of rain, barometric pressure and temperature); and because of these latter factors, on the season and on the time of day. Consequently, they vary very widely and some examples are given in Table 1. In remote areas and over the oceans, concentrations of mercury vapour are less than 1 ng/m^3; this is equivalent to less than 0·000001 ppm on a weight basis. In non-mineralised rural areas of the world regarded as 'unpolluted', atmospheric concentrations are usually in the range 1–10 ng/m^3; where copper-bearing deposits (in which mercury is present as an impurity) occur, concentrations may be rather higher, up to about 50 ng/m^3; where rocks are richest in mercury, e.g. where cinnabar deposits exist, levels up to 20,000 ng/m^3 have been recorded, but what proportion of this is due to mining activity is unknown; finally, in areas of volcanic activity, natural concentrations of 400–37,000 ng/m^3 and 730–40,700 ng/m^3 have been measured. (These levels approach the 'threshold limit value' (TLV) for industrial premises of 50 μg/m^3 (50,000 ng/m^3) (HMSO, 1973b); on a time-weighted basis, they actually exceed the TLV.) Quantities of mercury in air usually diminish with altitude and rain washes out both elemental and particulate mercury very effectively: even near mercury mines, concentrations after heavy rainstorms are almost zero (McCarthy et al, 1970).

A.53. There are few data available on atmospheric concentrations of mercury vapour in urban areas. In San Francisco, levels ranged from $0 \cdot 5$–50 ng/m^3 (Williston, 1968) and more recently a mean of 22 ng/m^3 (range up to 60 ng/m^3) was measured in Chicago (Wroblewski et al, 1974). Other recent work in the USA (Johnson and Braman, 1974; Braman and Johnson, 1974), in which a technique capable of analysing for volatile and particulate mercury and of distinguishing between a variety of volatile forms was used, has shown that mercury in air exists primarily (usually more than 90 per cent) in the volatile form, that the preponderance of the volatile mercury is in the elemental form and that other forms, e.g. methylmercuric compounds and mercuric salts were present. Total mercury concentrations ranged from $1 \cdot 8$–298 ng/m^3 at external sites and from 47–600 ng/m^3 inside buildings. Data for the UK are sparse, but in one industrial area the level away from known sources of mercury is typically <100 ng/m^3, whilst within a few hundred metres of a very large chloralkali works, mean levels of about 1,000 ng/m^3 have been observed.

A.54. There are also some data on particulate mercury in air, i.e. mercury associated with the solids present in air. In industrial areas of Europe, concentrations usually average about 3 ng/m^3, with peak levels up to about 15 ng/m^3; in residential areas, concentrations are usually less than 3 ng/m^3 but high values, similar to those observed in industrial areas, are sometimes observed – Table 1. The situation in the USA is similar. In the UK, rural areas exhibit concentrations of $0 \cdot 04$–$0 \cdot 20$ ng/m^3; data for urban areas are very sparse, but in the Swansea valley, concentrations range $<0 \cdot 01$–14 ng/m^3 (Table 1).

The hydrosphere

A.55. Mercury naturally present in the hydrosphere comes from volcanic activity, both via the atmosphere and directly, and from weathering processes. Man's industrial and (to a much lesser extent) agricultural practices also make a contribution.

Snow

A.56. Background levels of mercury in snow layers deposited in 800 BC average $0 \cdot 000062$ ppm – Table 2. Comparable levels have been observed in recent years in uncontaminated areas of Sweden, Canada and Greenland. It has been suggested (Weiss et al, 1971) that the higher concentrations (up to $0 \cdot 00023$ ppm) measured in Greenland snows deposited during the 1960s are a consequence of relatively recent increases in man's industrial use of mercury, with subsequent widespread dispersal. However, others (Carr and Wilkniss, 1973) have shown that high concentrations ($0 \cdot 000169$ ppm) exist in certain areas of Greenland in snows dating from 1870 and mentioned that this could possibly be a consequence of transport of mercury-containing volcanic ash from Iceland. It has also been suggested (Jonasson, 1973) that the presence of mercury (and other trace metals) in snow may sometimes be a consequence of upward migration of the metal, possibly by evaporation from underlying mineral deposits.

A.57. In urban areas, mercury concentrations in snow are usually less than 0·002 ppm, but near chloralkali plants in Sweden, levels up to 0·011 ppm have been recorded (Jernelov and Wallin, 1973).

Fresh water

A.58. Concentrations in rainwater in rural areas of the UK were recently measured as less than 0·0002 ppm – Table 2. Rather similar figures were given for Germany many years ago. Surface waters usually have only very low mercury concentrations, less than 0·00003 ppm, but on occasion up to 0·0002 ppm. Groundwaters have similar levels. There are very few data on mercury contamination of street surface run-off waters, although work in the USA has yielded a mean figure of 20 g of mercury per kilometre of street surface for mixed residential, industrial and commercial areas (Sartor et al, 1974).

A.59. River and estuary waters usually have very low levels of mercury. Published data (Table 2) show that the Test and Itchen have about 0·00001 ppm and that the Thames at its tidal limit has 0·000045 ppm. Unpublished data on rivers and canal waters, obtained in a co-operative survey between selected river authorities and the Department of the Environment, showed that 80 per cent of rivers sampled had levels of less than 0·001 ppm *total* mercury. This includes mercury associated with suspended solids. Other work (Smith et al, 1971) has shown that 82–98 per cent of mercury in water from the tidal reaches of the Thames is in particulate form, but the proportion associated with particulates may be rather lower in fresh waters. The harmonized monitoring scheme for UK waters (HMSO, 1974a) is now providing more data; thus the Tame in Lancashire varies from 0·00005–0·002 ppm, the Mersey from 0·00005–0·008 ppm and the Ribble is similar. In general, concentrations in un-contaminated rivers seem to be less than about 0·00005 ppm whereas major industrial rivers may have over 0·001 ppm. The situation in Europe and the USA is similar – Table 2. Sewage out-falls may contain high levels of mercury, up to about 0·003 ppm.

Estuarine and marine waters

A.60. Estuarine waters of the UK have mercury levels ranging from less than 0·00001 ppm to about 0·00025 ppm (Table 2), variations resulting from natural sources which influence background levels but more importantly from disposal of sewage sludges and industrial effluent. Again, most of the total mercury is associated with suspended solids. Coastal waters seem to be comparable over most of the globe, with mercury levels usually in the range 0·00001–0·0001 ppm except where industrial emissions occur. In Minimata Bay, Japan, up to 0·00066 ppm of mercury have been observed.

A.61. Ocean waters seem to vary considerably in mercury content. The North

55

Atlantic is reported to have levels of 0·000003–0·00002 ppm whereas the Ramapo Deep of the Pacific Ocean has 0·00008–0·00027 ppm mercury. Here, the concentration of mercury increases quite markedly with the depth of water. Recent work indicates that mean values range from 0·000011 ppm in the southern hemisphere to 0·000033 ppm in the northern hemisphere.

A.62. Most of the mercury reaching waters from industrial wastes is in the form of inorganic or organic compounds, whereas a high proportion of that reaching oceans from the air is in elemental form. The concentration of elemental mercury in water is limited to about 0·025 ppm by its solubility but in highly aerated waters the solubility may be substantially increased by the formation of chloride or carbonate complexes. In practice, it is unlikely that high mercury concentrations will be found because evaporation occurs from exposed surfaces and since most forms of mercury have a high affinity for organic substances, mercury is removed by aquatic organisms and by adsorption on sediments. Organic compounds of mercury can be biologically degraded to inorganic forms. The alkylmercury compounds are generally the most stable organic species and of these, the methylmercury compounds are the least biodegradable. Nevertheless, some de-methylation does occur.

The lithosphere

A.63. The lithosphere includes all crustal materials, e.g. soils, rocks and marine sediments (Table 3). The concentration of mercury in soils can be rather variable but is usually low. For the UK, an average of 0·060 ppm for some orchard soils (which are not necessarily typical of agricultural land in the UK) was found (Martin, 1963) and this is similar to levels for Sweden (0·060 ppm; Andersson, 1967), the Netherlands (0·090 ppm; Peolstra et al, 1973), Germany (0·070 ppm; Stock and Cucuel, 1934a) and the USA (0·070 ppm; Klein, 1972 and Shacklette et al, 1971). Although concentrations range up to about 1 ppm for agricultural soils, they are usually below about 0·2 ppm and the mean is below 0·1 ppm. Higher levels may occur in naturally mineralised areas, where up to 35 ppm has been observed, or where sewage sludges with a high mercury content have been spread, or where heavy doses of fungicides have been used over a long period.

A.64. Concentrations of mercury in rocks are similar to levels in soils. Both in sedimentary and igneous rocks, levels are usually below about 0·2 ppm (Table 3B), but there are exceptional areas, notably in the Crimea, where levels exist of up to 500 ppm, with a mean of 17 ppm. Deposits of mercury ore usually contain about 0·5–1·2 per cent mercury, i.e. 5,000–12,000 ppm. Other minerals often contain mercury as an impurity and some examples for northern Britain are given. The overall mean crustal concentration of mercury is estimated at about 0·070 ppm.

A.65. Mercury in sediments (Table 3C, D, E) has been widely studied, partially because sediments are laid down chronologically, thus apparently providing a historical pattern of concentrations back into the past, before the widespread use of mercury. In Lake Windermere, for instance, sediments dating from prior to the 19th century have levels below 0·3 ppm, whereas those dating from recent years show levels of about 1 ppm. This difference is usually attributed to contamination of recently-laid sediments by industrial mercury. However, it has been suggested (Sikes and Drain, 1973) that the activities and death of aquatic organisms would continually cycle mercury to the upper sediment layers; other authors (Aston et al, 1973) have mentioned the possibility that a geochemical mechanism would have the same result. Hence the existence of higher concentrations in upper layers may be at least in part a natural condition.

A.66. Sediments from rivers not known to be polluted usually have mercury concentrations of <0·1 ppm. However, downstream from emission sources such as chloralkali plants or paper mills some very much higher levels have been observed – Table 3. Sediments from major industrial rivers show a wide range of concentrations, typically 0·2–14 ppm for those in Europe. Sediments from tidal and estuarine regions show similar variations; those from unpolluted areas usually have mean levels of the order of 0·1 ppm but locally higher levels may exist.

A.67. Marine sediments also have higher concentrations in upper layers – Table 3E. Sediments in the Santa Barbara basin dating from 1,500 years ago have levels of about 0·04 ppm of mercury whereas those relating to the present have about 0·14 ppm mercury. The comments outlined above on whether this is a natural or man-induced phenomenon are also relevant here. Table 3E illustrates that levels of mercury found in the sediments of Minamata Bay were extremely high in comparison with levels in other areas regarded as polluted by man.

A.68. The importance of mercury in sediments lies in the fact that both inorganic and organic forms of mercury may be converted by natural processes to the highly toxic methylmercury form (Jensen and Jernelov, 1972). Two types of process are known: mercury-resistant bacteria with the ability to effect conversion under anaerobic conditions exist and enzymatic pathways have been described. (It has also been suggested that methylation of mercurials may occur by photolysis (Akagi and Takabatake, 1973), and via micro-organisms in soils and in the gut of animals and birds but no data yet convincingly support a methylating capacity in higher organisms (Krenkel, 1974)). At low concentrations of mercury, mainly dimethylmercury is formed, but at higher mercury concentrations, the monomethyl form predominates. The pH and oxygen content of the water are also important factors: a high pH favours formation of the dimethyl form, which decomposes to the monomethyl form at low pH, and methylation proceeds more efficiently under aerobic conditions. It has been estimated (Jernelov, 1972) that about 90–99 per cent of the mercury available in Earth's ecosystems is present in sediments, and of this proportion, 10 per cent may be in the methylmercury form. In contrast, less than 0·1 per cent is associated with the biosphere (most of this being in the non-methyl form, except in fish) and about 1–10 per cent, of which very little indeed is methylated, is probably present in the hydrosphere.

A.69. There are also a number of demethylating processes occurring in the environment and in various animals. Thus biological decomposition of methylmercury has been shown to occur in the presence of bacterial cultures and higher organisms after injection (Tonomura et al, 1968; Spangler et al, 1973), and dimethylmercury is converted into elemental mercury by ultra violet light.

A.70. Methylation is of importance because, being a natural process, it can affect all mercury emitted to water by man's activities. In addition, methylmercury compounds are readily absorbed but only very slowly excreted so are therefore accumulated by aquatic organisms. They are almost totally absorbed by the human alimentary tract and only very slowly excreted and are potentially the most hazardous form of mercury to man.

The biosphere

A.71. Data on the concentrations of mercury in terrestrial and aquatic vegetation and in terrestrial and aquatic animals have been previously summarised (Holden, 1972 and 1973; Kloke and Schenke, 1973).

A.72. *Terrestrial vegetation.* Typical soils that support vegetation contain very small amounts of inorganic mercury, usually <0·1 ppm (Table 3A) but it is not certain what proportion of this can be absorbed and translocated by the roots to the edible parts of the plant. However, analysis of plants grown on such soils (and not treated with mercurial compounds) suggests that mercury is not usually concentrated in the plant tissues. Thus levels usually range from about 0·001–0·2 ppm, with mean values usually <0·01 ppm but up to about 0·04 ppm. In the case of mushrooms and other edible fungi, some uptake does occur, leading to average concentrations of up to several ppm (Byrne et al, 1976; Frank et al, 1974; Stijve and Roschnik, 1974). For most plants, even when grown on soils having much higher concentrations of mercury, there is very little additional uptake. Thus it was found that all the edible portions of vegetables, with the exception of onions, had levels of <0·1 ppm when grown on soils experimentally treated to contain up to 10 ppm of mercury. Some uptake did occur, but not into edible parts of crops (Bache et al, 1973). Other work, involving plants grown in soil regularly treated with sewage sludge rich in mercury, showed that plants took up only a very small proportion of the additional mercury (van Loon, 1974) and this proportion has been estimated to be about one-hundredth of the total present (Andersson and Nilsson, 1972). Unpublished work of this type has similarly shown that vegetables took up <0·01 ppm of mercury from sludge-treated soils containing up to 5·4 ppm of mercury. Finally, plants grown downwind from a mercury emission source (a power plant) have been shown (Klein and Russell, 1973) to contain quantities of mercury similar to those observed in local background areas, despite the fact that the soil on which they were growing was clearly contaminated.

A.73. The fate of mercurial plant pesticides varies according to the crop to which they are applied, the particular compound used, areas and methods of application, dosage levels and pre-harvest intervals. The greatest use of mercury in the UK, for the treatment of cereal seeds, has very little effect on mercury levels in the grain produced. And Canadian work (Saha et al, 1970) indicates that treated seed containing 12–16 ppm of mercury yielded grain with residues of only 0·008–0·016 ppm; other work (Selikoff, 1971) showed levels in the grain of up to 0·1 ppm; clearly there is little transfer. Similarly, in the case of foliar spraying of fruit trees, only a little transfer takes place. The application takes place at pre-blossom and early growth stages and a six-week harvesting interval is prescribed. Average levels in the fruit have not usually exceeded 0·070 ppm (range up to 0·36 ppm), while background levels are usually in the region of 0·005–0·04 ppm.

A.74. *Aquatic vegetation.* Concentrations of mercury in aquatic plants are usually much higher than in the water in which they live; thus 0·030–0·037 ppm was found in seaweeds living in water with only 0·00003 ppm (Stock and Cucuel, 1934a). Aquatic plants can take up mercury by adsorption on the surface of submerged parts, the amount of uptake varying with species: fresh-water plants sampled above a paper mill discharging mercurial effluent had concentrations of about 0·08 ppm whereas those sampled downstream had about 37 ppm of mercury (Johnels et al, 1967). Water plants sampled close to chloralkali works in Bavaria have been found with mercury concentrations as high as 295 ppm (*dry* weight) (Schramel et al, 1973). There is little or no information on mercury levels in plants living in water naturally rich in mercury.

A.75. Mercury compounds may be toxic to phytoplankton species at very low concentrations. As little as 0·00006 ppm of phenylmercury acetate in water has been shown to inhibit the growth of three species of phytoplankton, and maximum inhibition was observed at concentrations of 0·003 ppm and above. Mercuric chloride is much less toxic (Nuzzi, 1972).

A.76. *Aquatic animals.* Mercury concentrations in aquatic creatures have been reviewed by Holden (1972; 1973). The members of aquatic food chains include dissolved substances, phyto- and zooplankton, insects, crustacea, small and large fish and aquatic mammals. Zooplankton were reported to have a mean concentration of about 0·14 ppm in an unpolluted area. Mercury is transported through food chains following uptake from the medium (water, sediment) by bacteria, phytoplankton etc. and subsequently by one species feeding on another at a lower trophic level. The most important concentration step for mercury is at the initial medium to organism transfer. In very general terms, concentrations in creatures might be expected to increase as one moves up the food chain to the larger predators, but the situation is confused by a lack of studies where a specific food chain is followed and by the fact that increasing age of the sampled species often leads to increasing concentration.

A.77. Early analyses of freshwater fish for mercury gave levels of 0·03–0·18 ppm (Stock and Cucuel, 1934a) and 0·076–0·167 ppm (Raeder and Snekvik, 1940). Much more recent analyses continue to yield comparable results, e.g. Johnels et al (1967) found 0·06–0·14 ppm in pike living in waters believed free

F

from pollution arising from human activities. However, much higher levels have been observed in this species living in contaminated waters. In general, slight contamination may lead to levels of 0·1–0·3 ppm; moderate contamination, such as that occurring upstream from a pulp mill using mercurial fungicides, may lead to levels of 0·25–1·5 ppm; and excessive contamination, such as that existing downstream from such a pulp mill may produce levels approaching 10 ppm in pike (Holden, 1972).

A.78. A number of other species of freshwater fish have been examined in many areas of the world. The same basic conclusions may be drawn; namely that levels up to about 0·2 ppm exist in uncontaminated waters and may thus be regarded as natural, but that much higher levels, up to several ppm, exist in polluted areas. Of particular interest are the data for fish from the Agano River, Niigata, where the second outbreak of Minamata disease occurred. Here, levels in fish were found to be up to 23 ppm (Holden, 1972).

A.79. Relatively high concentrations (i.e. close to or greater than 0·5 ppm, the current USA Food and Drugs Administration acceptable limit) are sometimes observed for certain predatory fish living in unpolluted water. Thus bass in a reservoir in the USA contained up to 0·74 ppm of mercury (Knight and Herring, 1972). Here, as in many other studies, a positive correlation was established between fish size (and thus age) and mercury concentration.

A.80. Holden (1972; 1973) has also summarised the data for marine fish. The typical range for fish from unpolluted waters is about 0·01–0·2 ppm (wet weight), but even more restricted in certain cases, e.g. 0·013–0·026 ppm for Greenland cod. Levels observed today in unpolluted areas are not different from those observed 40 years ago in comparable areas (Stock and Cucuel, 1934a). Higher levels are again observed in certain localities known to be polluted, e.g. up to 3·1 ppm in plaice at Oresund, Sweden, and up to 2·5 ppm in some coastal fish off the UK. In the latter case the mean values were 0·45–0·64 ppm. In contrast, fish taken from the restricted waters of Minamata Bay had very high levels of mercury, up to 50 ppm.

A.81. For some marine fish, as for freshwater fish, relatively high levels (greater than 0·5 ppm) are observed. Thus tuna, swordfish, blue marlin, black marlin and halibut have all been found with high levels of mercury (Kamps et al,1972; Rivers et al, 1972; Mackay et al, 1975; Simpson et al, 1974). It is important to establish whether this is a natural phenomenon or a consequence of industrial pollution and examinations of museum specimens have been used in attempts to answer this point. In one study (Miller et al, 1972), it was found that seven museum specimens of tuna, dating from 1878 to 1909, had mercury concentrations in the range 0·26–0·64 ppm and one swordfish dating from 1946 had 0·52 ppm. Recent specimens of tuna had levels of 0·13–0·48 ppm and recent swordfish had 0·23–1·27 ppm of mercury. In another study (Barber et al, 1972), it was noted that the mercury concentration of bottom-dwelling fish depended primarily on size and species, and the levels in a museum specimen caught 90 years ago fitted closely the size-concentration regression curve established for nine recently-caught individuals of the same species. Similar observations have been made for some long-lived freshwater fish (Sumner et al, 1972).

A.82. In contrast, a study of many species of freshwater fish from the Great Lakes has shown that only five out of 57 preserved specimens, taken between 1938 and 1939, contained mercury in excess of 0·5 ppm (Evans et al, 1972). A more recent study (Gibbs et al, 1974) of marine fish has indicated that preservation procedures and the passage of time may influence levels of metal residues in fish.

A.83. Shellfish are known to be able to concentrate a number of metals to a considerable degree and so even those living in unpolluted waters may themselves contain relatively high levels. Thus Johnels et al (1967) found 0·14 ppm in freshwater crayfish and Holden and Topping (1972) found levels of 0·12–0·75 ppm in lobsters. In contrast, molluscs from Minamata Bay were found to contain 11–40 ppm of mercury (quoted in Holden, 1973).

A.84. Fish living in moderately polluted areas and containing relatively high concentrations of mercury rarely seem to suffer in consequence any significant biological effect. (There is evidence that the element selenium, which is also accumulated by some aquatic life, may have a protective effect against the toxic action of mercury (Koeman et al, 1973).) However, in extreme circumstances, e.g. at Minamata Bay, fish and shell-fish contained 9–24 ppm of mercury and many of these were dead. The 48 hour LC_{50} (the concentration expressed as mg/l* (equal to ppm on a weight basis) of mercuric chloride in sea water killing 50 per cent of the subjects in 48 hours) for various marine species ranges from 0·075–10 mg/l (ppm) (Portmann and Wilson, 1971). The half-life of mercury in fish is about 110 days. Much longer half-lives, up to about 1,000 days in the case of the eel, have also been observed.

A.85. Perhaps the most important feature of mercury in fish is that the great majority is present as methylmercury, the most toxic form of mercury. This occurs because many forms of mercury are converted by bacteria in sediments to methylmercury and this, having a high affinity for proteins and being fat-soluble, is most readily absorbed from food but not readily excreted by fish. The links in this transfer are not fully understood. For fish, the proportion of total mercury present in the methylmercury form is usually given as 85–95 per cent (Holden, 1973); in shellfish, the proportion is rather more variable, ranging from 40–90 per cent (HMSO, 1971).

A.86. There are also some data on seals living around the coast of UK (Hepplestone and French, 1973). These animals showed highest mercury levels in the liver, intermediate levels in the kidneys and lower levels in the brain. Distinct regional differences were observed: thus mean liver concentrations (fresh weight) reached 113 ppm in seals from the Outer Hebrides, but were only 4·9 ppm in those from the Shetlands. Brain levels were 0·7 ppm and 0·3 ppm respectively. Seals from East Anglia, the Farne Islands and West Scotland

*1 mg/l is 1 milligram/litre.

showed intermediate levels, other data (Holden, in the press) indicates liver concentrations up to 720 ppm (fresh weight) and brain levels up to 16·8 ppm. As far as is known, these levels have no effect upon the seals.

A.87. *Terrestrial animals*. Most attention in this area has been given to mercury in the seed-eating and fish-eating birds of Sweden, primarily because it was in these cases that the first suspicions concerning the environmental effects of mercury arose. There is now little doubt that mercury concentrations in certain forms of terrestrial Swedish wildlife have increased since the pre-industrial era, and here examinations of museum specimens have proved useful. Berg et al (1966) showed that mercury levels in falcons' tail feathers increased from 2·5 ppm for the period 1834–1940 to values over 40 ppm for the period 1941–1965. Similar observations have been made for eagle-owls, white-tailed eagles and goshawks. More recent work (Borg et al, 1969) has reported concentrations of 0·03–200 ppm (dry weight) in livers of birds which died and 3–11 ppm in unhatched eggs. Usually, more than 75 per cent of the mercury present was in the form of methylmercury. Following discontinuation of the use of alkyl-mercury seed treatments and of mercury in the paper and pulp industry in Sweden, there has been some evidence of decreasing mercury levels in terrestrial wildlife (Emmelin, 1974; Westermark et al, 1975) and also in samples of northern pike (Olsson, 1976).

A.88. A similar picture has emerged from Canadian work. Birds from Saskatchewan were shown to contain lower mercury levels than birds from Alberta, where much more widespread use of alkylmercury seed treatments occurred (Fimreite et al, 1970); and high levels were observed in grebes from Pinchi Lake, near a mercury mine, and in cormorants and herons from coastal waters (quoted in Holden, 1972).

A.89. Data are also available for birds living near the Scottish coast (Dale et al, 1973). Eiders, which feed largely on mussels, had mercury levels in the liver of 24–48 ppm (dry weight) but the livers of estuarine fish feeders contained the highest levels, up to 122 ppm (dry weight) in one case. Pelagic sea-birds had lower levels (less than 10 ppm dry weight), as did gulls from oceanic islands. The lowest level amongst sea birds was found in a guillemot, 0·7 ppm (dry weight). Three samples of terrestrial birds had 2–28 ppm mercury (dry weight) in their livers. More extensive work (Parslow et al, 1972), found that puffins from around the coast of northern England and Scotland had levels of mercury in their livers ranging from 2·8–7·7 ppm (dry weight), with a mean of 2·16 ppm (dry) for mercury in their eggs. Mean mercury concentrations in guillemot eggs from Lundy, Skomer and Berry Head were found to be 5·35, 4·61 and 6·25 ppm dry weight respectively, whilst the level in kittiwake eggs from the same areas were rather lower at 1·73, 1·45 and 2·32 ppm dry weight respectively (Parslow, 1973a).

A.90. Mercury levels were also measured in gannets found dead in unusually large numbers on the east and west coasts of Britain in 1972. Liver concentrations ranged from 5·9 ppm to 52·7 ppm with one bird having an exceptionally high level of 97·7 ppm (dry weight); most were below 25 ppm. Concentrations were higher in gannets from the Irish Sea than in those from the Firth of Forth and data from other species and from eggs are consistent with this finding (Parslow et al, 1973). Other data (Holdgate, 1971; Tejning, 1967) suggest that mercury may have contributed to death in the exceptional cases.

A.91. Recently, data have been reported for wading birds living in the Wash (Parslow, 1973b). Mercury levels in the liver of the knot were observed to change seasonally, increasing from a minimum of about 0·3–0·4 ppm (wet) in early autumn to a maximum in late winter (February/March) up to 20 times higher, i.e. 6–8 ppm (wet). This may be a consequence of migration patterns, the former birds having spent the summer on the east coast, whereas the latter birds come from mainland Europe, having spent the autumn in the Wadden Sea. There was no evidence of any harmful physiological effects associated with the higher levels, but it was suggested that since the Wash is relatively unpolluted by industrial mercury, wading birds elsewhere, e.g. in industrialised estuaries, might be at risk.

A.92. Wild birds, such as wood pigeons, and game birds have also been examined. Following incidents in which large numbers of wild birds were found dead or dying in the East Lothian area, the East Craigs Laboratory of the Department of Agriculture and Fisheries for Scotland (DAFS) surveyed in 1972 and 1973 the pesticide contents (including mercury) of tissues from such birds. Levels of mercury (wet weight) in the breast and liver tissues of wood pigeons ranged from 0·02–0·53 ppm and 0·04–10·1 ppm respectively, and in pinkfoot geese 0·1–0·4 ppm and 2·2–8·4 ppm respectively. It was concluded that mortality was probably connected with the difficult sowing conditions prevailing at the time, allowing undue access to the treated seed by wildlife, leading to enhanced consumption of mercury and also of dieldrin, the latter probably being responsible for death. A number of birds were also shot in East Lothian during 1972 and 1973. In this case, the level of mercury (again wet weight) in breast tissues of wood pigeons showed an overall mean of 0·04 ppm (range <0·01–0·17 ppm) in the late summer/early autumn of 1972, a mean of 0·09 ppm (range <0·01–0·72 ppm) at the turn of the year (1972/73), rising to a mean of 0·43 ppm (range 0·06–1·22 ppm) in spring 1973 and falling again to a mean of 0·03 ppm (range <0·01–0·18 ppm) in summer 1973. The bodies of these birds and also of living field mice, which in the two months following sowing of treated seed can contain up to 37 μg of mercury (Jefferies and French, 1976) form obvious sources of mercury for predatory mammals and birds. However, recent measurements of mercury residues in a large sample of British barn and tawny owls (Stanley and Elliott, 1976) have demonstrated mean total mercury residue levels of 0·25 ppm and 0·18 ppm (wet weight) respectively in pectoral muscle. These levels are considerably lower than those in the same species in Sweden and the Netherlands.

A.93. Data on terrestrial animals other than birds has also been collected (Holden, 1972). In Sweden, carnivorous animals generally contained higher mercury levels than herbivorous animals and in Canada, regional differences between animals in Alberta and in Saskatchewan have been observed. Mercury levels in man are discussed in Chapter 3.

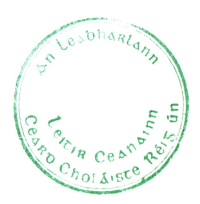

APPENDIX II

COMPOSITION OF THE WORKING GROUP

Chairman:

T. P. Hughes, Deputy Secretary (Environmental Protection), Department of the Environment.

Deputy Chairman:

A. J. Fairclough, Director, Central Unit on Environmental Pollution, Department of the Environment.

Technical Secretary:

J. P. Giltrow, Central Unit on Environmental Pollution, Department of the Environment.

Departments represented:

Cabinet Office (CO).
Department of Agriculture and Fisheries for Scotland (DAFS).
Department of Education and Science (DES).
Department of the Environment (DOE).
Department of Health and Social Security (DHSS).
Department of Industry (DI).
Department of Prices and Consumer Protection (DPCP).
Health and Safety Executive (HSE).
Home Office (HO).
Ministry of Agriculture, Fisheries and Food (MAFF).
Scottish Development Department (SDD).
Scottish Home and Health Department (SHHD).
Welsh Office (WO).

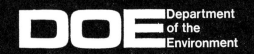

Press Notice 795

25th October 1974

DOE REGISTER OF RESEARCH

The Department of the Environment has set up a new data bank of recently-completed and ongoing UK research projects in subjects relating to the Department's interests together with a free enquiry service giving access to the information. The Register is intended for the use of research workers, institutions, organisations commissioning research and planning research programmes, and the professions.

The Register of Research – covering construction, planning, pollution, environment, resources, transport and roads – has been established by co-ordinating and expanding several surveys formerly carried out by or on behalf of the Department.

Data on the Register for each project gives details of where the research is being done, the title and a short description, names of the research workers, sponsorship and finance, the start and expected completion dates, and a list of any publications arising from the research. Information on the Register will be updated annually.

The Register operates from three centres, each responsible for specific subject areas as follows:

For Building and Construction Research:
Library (RR)
Building Research Establishment
Garston
Watford
Herts.
WD2 7JR
Telephone: Garston (Herts.) 74040 ext 442. Telex 923229

For Planning, Pollution, Environment and Resources Research:
  DOE Library (Research) P3/173
  2 Marsham Street
  London
  SW1P 3EB
  Telephone: 01-212 4328. Telex 22801

For Transportation and Road Research:
  Technical Information and Library Services
  Transport and Road Research Laboratory
  Crowthorne
  Berks.
  RG11 6AU
  Telephone: Crowthorne 3131. Telex 848272

The Register may be consulted by post, telephone, telex or by visit by appointment at the appropriate centres which will also handle enquiries cutting across subject areas.

A print-out entitled 'DOE Register of Research 1974' of the projects held on the Register in the first half of 1974 may be obtained free of charge from the appropriate centre in the fields of Construction (Part I – available in December 1974) and Environmental Planning (Part II – available now). For 1975 additional parts are planned including Part III on Transport and Part IV on Environmental Pollution.

Note to editors

The DOE Register of Research replaces a number of regular priced publications such as the Survey of Research and Development for the Construction Industry (last published by HMSO in 1972) and the Register of Planning Research produced by the Royal Town Planning Institute. The latter's last publication entitled 'Environmental Planning Research' is available from the Reader Services Librarian, Room C3/01, Headquarters Library, DOE, 2 Marsham Street, London SW1 3EB, price £5. It relates to work in progress or completed in 1973.
Telephone No.: 01-212 3434.
Night Calls (6.30 p.m. to 8.00 a.m.)
Weekends and Holidays:
01-212 7071.

TABLE 1

Mercury in the atmosphere

A. Remote and rural areas

Location	Concentration, ng/m³	Comment	Reference
Northern Norway	<0·005–0·06, mean <0·015	remote area, particulate	Heindryckx et al, 1973
Jungfraujoch (Swiss Alps)	0·025		
Over the Pacific Ocean	0·6–0·7 (vapour)	20 miles off San Francisco	Williston, 1968
Dourbes (remote area of Ardennes)	0·4±0·2	particulate	Heindryckx et al, 1973
Houffalize (village in Ardennes)	0·3±0·2		
Zeebrugge (sea coast)	usually <0·2 but up to ca 2		
Germany	8	regarded as unpolluted air	Stock and Cucuel, 1934b
Pala Alto, California	1–10	vapour	Goldwater and Clarkson, 1972
Non-mineralised areas of USA	3–9 (vapour)	sampled at 400 ft elevation	McCarthy et al, 1970
Near copper deposits in USA	7–53	ditto	
Niles, Michigan (rural)	1·9	particulate	Dams et al, 1970
Iceland	400–37,000	near areas of volcanic activity	Siegel et al, 1973
Hawaii	730–40,700; mean 26,000	near areas of volcanic activity	Siegel et al, 1973b
Hawaii	ca 20	as particulate only in the dilute fume	Cadle et al, 1973
Various regions of UK	0·04–0·20	data for seven sites, particulate	Peirson et al, 1973
World-wide	20	estimated world average	Eriksson, 1967

Total global flux of mercury from continents to atmosphere as a consequence of natural processes estimated as 25,000–150,000 tonnes/annum (Weiss et al, 1971).

B. Urban areas

Location	Concentration, ng/m³	Comment	Reference
Europe			
Ghent, Antwerp, Liege	2–15, mean ca 3	industrial plant in area ⎱ particulate	Heindryckx et al, 1973
Ghent, Antwerp, Brussels, Liege, Charleroi, Mechelen	usually < 3 but up to 19	residential areas ⎰	
Finland, urban	0·2		quoted in Hasanen, 1973
Heidelberg	0·02–0·42, mean 0·17		Bogen, 1973
Paris	11·2		quoted in Bogen, 1973
Swansea, Neath, Port Talbot	range < 0·01–14	particulate	Welsh Office, 1975
USA			
Chicago	10 ⎱	particulate, 1946–1951	Cholak, 1952
Cincinnati	30–210, mean 100 ⎰		
Charleston	170		
New York	1–14 outdoor / 1–41 indoor, offices, laboratories ⎰	particulate	Jones, 1971
San Francisco	0·5–25 in winter ⎱ vapour / 1·5–50 in summer ⎰		Williston, 1968
East Chicago	4·8	particulate	Dams et al, 1970
Dallas	5–5680 ⎱ vapour / 3	homes, offices, laboratories / background	Foote, 1972

69

Location	Concentration, ng/m³	Comment	Reference
Buffalo, New York	1–30	particulate	Pillay et al, 1972
Chicago metropolitan area	3–39	particulate	Brar et al, 1969
Chicago	2–10 (mean 4)	particulate	Wroblewski et al, 1974
	5–60 (mean 22)	vapour	
St. Louis	0·42, downtown 0·26, 20 miles downwind	particulate	Tanner et al, 1974
	0·05, 40 miles downwind 0·12, 60 miles downwind		
Toronto, Canada	0·14–0·35		de Geoij and Houtman, 1971
C. Industrial			
In chlor-alkali plants	up to 100,000	vapour	Friberg, 1951
In thermometer and electrical workshops	100,000–290,000 usually 6–290, but up to 1,600,000 at bench surfaces today's levels approx. 35,000	vapour	Bidstrup et al, 1951
In university facilities	10,000–35,000 peaks over 50,000	vapour	Mayz et al, 1971
Near base-metal and precious metal mines	ca 25	sampled at 400 ft.	McCarthy et al, 1970
	68–1,500	sampled at ground	
Near mercury mines	24–108	sampled at 400 ft.	
	2,000–20,000	sampled at ground	

70

Location	Concentration, ng/m³	Comment	Reference
Within mercury mines	up to 2,000,000	} vapour	Neville, 1967
	up to 5,000,000		Jones, 1971
Threshold limit values	50,000	all forms except alkyl compounds	} HMSO, 1973b
	10,000	alkyl compounds	
Saturation concentration of vapour at 17°C	1,000,000	does not take particulates into account	Jenne, 1970

71

TABLE 2

Mercury in the hydrosphere

Location and type	Concentration, ppm	Reference
Rainwater		
Rural UK sites	<0·0002	Peirson et al, 1973
Germany	0·00005–0·00048, mean of 0·0002	Stock and Cucuel, 1934a
Drinking water		
Loch Kirbister	<0·00001 (detection limit)	Private communication (DAFS)
Various reservoirs in Germany	<0·00003	quoted in Bouquiaux, 1973
Purified surface waters in Netherlands, Germany, Luxembourg	usually <0·00003, but up to 0·0002	ditto
Spring and well waters, Germany	0·00001–0·00005	Stock and Cucuel, 1934a
Tap, spring and reservoir water, Yugoslavia	0·0001–0·0002, 0·0003 and 0·00011 respectively	quoted in Holden, 1972
Mains water, Germany (Mainz)	0–0·013, mean 0·00084	quoted in Bouquiaux, 1973
Groundwaters		
Netherlands, Germany	usually <0·0001, but up to 0·00022	quoted in Bouquiaux, 1973
Finland	0·0002	quoted in Hasanen, 1973
Snow layers		
Sweden: surface layer	0·00007	} Johnels et al, 1967
sublayer	0·00021	
Sweden: background	0·00008–0·00012	} Jernelov and Wallin, 1973
near chloralkali plant	usually <0·002, but up to 0·011	

Location and type	Concentration, ppm	Reference
Canada: urban (Ottawa)	0·0035–0·004 (1971) 0·000065–0·000123 (1972)	Jonasson, 1973
rural, unmineralised area	<0·00001	
rural, mineralised area	0·00001–0·00052	
Greenland	0·000062 (800 BC) 0·000030–0·000066 (19th century) 0·000087–0·00023 (1960s)	Weiss et al, 1971
Greenland: site 1	0·000013 (1850 AD) 0·000050 (1940 AD)	Carr and Wilkniss, 1973
site 2	0·000169 (1870 AD) 0·000100 (1930 AD)	
Antarctica	0·000075 (1724 AD)	Weiss et al, 1971
Rivers and estuaries		
UK		
River Test, River Itchen	0·00001	Leatherland et al, 1971
River Thames: Teddington Gravesend Sewage effluent outfall	0·000045 } 82–98 per cent in 0·00040 } particulate form 0·0029	Smith et al, 1971
Solent and English Channel	0·000011–0·000021	Burton and Leatherland, 1971
Severn Estuary; Cardiff Central Bristol Channel	ca 0·00005 } in solution <0·00001 }	Gardner and Riley, 1973a
Cardiff Central Bristol Channel	>0·0002 } particulate ca 0·0001 }	

73

Location and type	Concentration, ppm	Reference
Forth Estuary: at Forth Bridge further upstream	0·00013–0·00016 up to 0·00025	Private communication (DAFS)
Tay Estuary, sewage outfalls	0·00003–0·00207	
Sweden		
Unpolluted Contaminated	0·00004 0·00027–0·00051	Hasselrot, 1968
Unpolluted Contaminated (Stockholm Archipelago)	0·00013 0·00025	Johnels et al, 1967
USA		
Geological survey showed: 34 rivers 27 rivers 10 rivers 2 rivers	<0·0001 0·0001–0·001 0·001–0·005 >0·005	Wershaw, 1970
Detroit river	0·03	quoted in Holden, 1972
Savannah estuary	up to 0·00045	Windom, 1973
USSR		
European rivers Armenian rivers and lake	0·0004–0·0028, mean 0·0011 0·001–0·003	quoted in Wershaw, 1970
Europe		
Germany: River Saale River Elbe River Rhine	0·000035–0·000145 0·00009 0·001–0·003; 0·001	Heide et al, 1957 Kempf, 1973; Stock and Cucuel, 1934a

Location and type	Concentration, ppm	Reference
Italy: uncontaminated near mercury deposit Rivers Raglia, Fiora River Albegna	0·00001–0·00005 up to 0·136 usually <0·000001 exceptionally up to 0·021	Dall'Aglio, 1968 Bombace et al, 1973
Bavaria	<0·00001–0·0018	Schramel et al, 1973
General: 'pure' river waters less pure rivers (e.g. Weser, Rhine, Maas, Scheldt, Yser, Thames)	0–0·0005, mean 0·00015 usually 0·0004–0·0007, up to 0·003	quoted in Bouquiaux, 1973
Japan	<0·00001–0·0001	Holden, 1972
Marine waters		
Southern Irish Sea	0·00003–0·00005 in solution <0·00002 particulate	Gardner and Riley, 1973a
Irish Sea: surface waters excluding coastal strip central area eastern coastal strip	0·000025–0·000050, mean 0·000032 0·00001–0·000024, mean 0·000018 >0·0002 (up to 0·0009)	Gardner and Riley, 1973b
Waddenzee (Netherlands)	ca 0·00015	Bouquiaux, 1973
North Sea (Heligoland)	0·00003	Stock and Cucuel, 1934a
North Atlantic	0·000003–0·000020	quoted in Fitzgerald and Lyons, 1973
Various areas, covering the following range: S.W. Indian Ocean Subtropical N. Atlantic Ocean	0·000011, mean 0·000033, mean	Gardner, 1975
Canadian continental shelf waters Greenland Sea	0·000058–0·000071 0·000016–0·000364	quoted in Fitzgerald and Lyons, 1973 ditto
North Sea and outer Moray Firth	0·00001–0·00005	Topping and Pirie, 1972

75

Location and type	Concentration, ppm	Reference
USA, coastal waters	0·000045–0·000078, total 0·000021–0·000033, inorganic 0·00014–0·000050, organic	Fitzgerald and Lyons, 1973
USA, coastal waters off Georgia	0·00001–0·0003, usually <0·0001	Windom, 1973
Pacific Ocean, Ramapo Deep (south-east of Honshu)	0·00008–0·00015 at surface 0·00006–0·00024 at 500 m 0·00015–0·00027 at 3,000 m	Hosohara, 1961
Minamata Bay, Japan	0·00008–0·00066	Hosohara et al, 1961
Waters of USSR	0·0007–0·002	quoted in Wershaw, 1970
Thermal waters		
From hot springs, USA From hot springs, USSR	0–0·0015 0·0005–0·004	White et al, 1970
Total flux of mercury from continents to oceans by natural weathering is variously given as:	230 tonnes/annum 800 tonnes/annum 2,500 tonnes/annum 3,000 tonnes/annum 3,800 tonnes/annum 5,000 tonnes/annum	Joensuu, 1971 Gavis and Ferguson, 1972 de Geoij and Houtman, 1971 Peakall and Lovett, 1972 Weiss et al, 1971 Goldberg, 1968; Goldberg and Gross, 1971

The total flux of mercury from sub-marine floor to oceans from sub-marine volcanic activity has not been estimated but seems likely to be substantial

TABLE 3

Mercury in the lithosphere

Location and type	Concentration, ppm	Remarks	Reference
A. SOILS			
European soils, various	0·100 0·010	at surface at 100 cm deep	⎱ Frissell et al, 1973
Rural areas From bulb growing areas	<0·100 ca 0·15	at surface in upper layers	⎰
Foreland soils	up to 12		
Soils, various collected values	0·005–5·0, mean 0·10		Kloke and Schenke, 1973
Finnish soils	0·020 0·200 0·130	unpolluted contaminated peat	⎱ quoted in Hasanen, 1973
Scottish soils: Agricultural areas	0·010–0·76, usually <0·20 0·13–1·0 0·06–0·89 0·06–0·23	medium loams clay loams sand, sandy loams peaty loams	⎱ DAFS (unpublished)
Non-agricultural areas	0·06–1·96, usually <0·40		
English	0·01–0·06	normal	Martin, 1963
	0·25–15	natural geological origin	Warren and Delavault, 1969
Sweden	0·018 ± 0·001	topsoil	⎱ Andersson and Nilsson, 1972
	ca 0·675	after adding mercury- containing sludge for 12 years	⎰

Location and type	Concentration, ppm	Remarks	Reference
Sweden	0·001–0·029 0·030–0·034 } Mean 0·070 0·10–0·29 0·14–1·0	sand clays forest soils cultivated soils	Stock and Cucuel, 1934a
British Columbia	0·05–0·25 exceptionally up to 2·0 1–10	near gold, molybdenum and base metal deposits near mercury deposits	Warren and Delavault, 1969
Saskatchewan	0·011–0·060 0·005–0·057	cultivated soils uncultivated soils	Gracey and Stewart, 1974
California	0·02–0·04	background	Fleischer, 1970
	0·38 278	unmineralised areas mineralised areas	Jonasson, 1973
Winconsin	0·03–0·3	background level	Syers et al, 1973
Japan	0·33 0·33 } means 0·28 0·18	paddy fields ordinary fields orchard soils forest soils	Environment Agency, 1975
Eastern shore soils	0·008 0·010	background enriched	Klein and Russell, 1973
Idrija, Yugoslavia	0·54–0·56 4·7 11·5–35·1	background 5 km from mercury mine in ore-bearing area	Stegner et al 1973
Northern California	up to 500	muds from volcanic regions	White et al, 1970

Location and type	Concentration, ppm	Remarks	Reference
B. ROCKS			
General			
Igneous – granites etc.	usually <0·20 average <0·10	wide variations occur	Fleischer, 1970
Exceptionally, e.g. in Crimea and Donets Basin	up to 500 with a mean of ca 17		
Metamorphic	means range 0·018–0·407	wide variations occur	
Sedimentary			
Limestones, sandstones, shales and clays	usually <0·20 average 0·03–0·05	wide variations	
	exceptionally up to a mean of 5–6	Crimea	
Mercury ore (cinnabar)	5,000–12,000 = 0·5–1·2 per cent	Spain	
Northern Britain: minerals			
Lead ores (galena)	0·04–0·9, exceptionally up to 47		DAFS (unpublished)
Zincblende ores	4–15		
Cuprous manganese	1·8–3		
Malachite	6·5		
Linarite, pyromorphite, scheelite, chalcopyrite, mica	0·03–0·5		
Sandstones	0·01–2·5, mean ca 0·05–0·08		
Overall crustal mean concentration is estimated at about 0·070 ppm			

Location and type	Concentration, ppm	Remarks	Reference
C. SEDIMENTS			
1. Freshwater sediments			
Lake Windermere	1·026, mean 0·680 0·286 0·122	20th century ⎱ muds 19th century ⎰ 15th-18th century ⎱ brown 520-1400 AD ⎰ clay	Aston et al, 1973
Lake Michigan	0·06-0·09 (wet)	background	Syers et al, 1973
Lake in Wisconsin	0·01-0·24 (wet)	precultural times	
River Dart above tidal limit	0·01-0·42, mean 0·07 (dry)		Taylor, 1973
Rivers Paglia, Fiora and Albegna, Italy	usually <0·10 but up to 70 in polluted areas		Bombace et al, 1973
Mississippi river	0·08-0·57	Proportion of methyl mercury was 0·01-0·07 per cent	Andren and Harriss, 1973
Bavarian rivers	0·10-4·6 (dry) but up to 112 downstream of factory		Schramel et al, 1973
Swedish rivers	0·034-0·168 (dry) up to 18·4 below paper mill 11·6-26·5 below chloralkali plant		Hasselrot, 1968
Sediments from drinking water reservoirs in Germany and Luxembourg	0-1, mean 0·020	unpolluted	Bouquiaux, 1973
Sediments from Rivers Maas, Scheldt, Yser, Grindstedt	mean ca 0·25, but up to 3·62	dry, contaminated polluted area	

Location and type	Concentration, ppm	Remarks	Reference
Lake Erie	0·50–12·4 (dry)	polluted	Pillay et al, 1972
Lake Michigan	0·03–0·38 (dry)		Kennedy et al, 1971
Rivers Danube, Rhine, Ems, Weser and Elbe	0·2–14		Kloke and Schenke, 1973
Finland	0·05 ⎫ dry 1·0–170 ⎭	unpolluted polluted	Hasanen, 1973

2. Tidal river and estuarial sediments

Location and type	Concentration, ppm	Remarks	Reference
River Tawe	0·15 at top 0·31 at 1 in. deep 0·76 at 6 in. deep ⎫		
River Neath	0·15 at 1 in. deep 0·16 at 6 in. deep	dry	
Shore at University College, Swansea	0·045 at top 0·040 at 6 in. deep		Bloxam et al, 1972
Blackpill	0·100 at top 0·140 at 6 in. deep		
Swansea Bay, West Pier	0·090 at top 0·090 at 6 in. deep ⎭		
Swansea Bay	0·02–1·6 (dry)		Clifton and Vivian, 1975
Dart Estuary Dartmouth	0·01–0·55, mean 0·22 <0·01–0·26, mean 0·05 ⎱ dry		⎱ Taylor, 1973
River Wyre	0·04–8·5, mean 3·3	mud, top 2 cm ⎫	⎫
River Mersey	0·40–6·0, mean 3·4	⎬ dry	⎬ Private communication (MAFF)
River Dee	0·02 0·80–1·3	sand mud ⎭	⎭

81

Location and type	Concentration, ppm	Remarks	Reference
River Mersey	<0·01–14·30, mean 2·23 (dry)		Craig and Morton, 1976
Everglades, Florida	0·12–0·49 (total)	0·01–0·07 per cent present as methylmercury	Andren and Harriss, 1973
Savannah river, USA (salt marsh)	0·10–0·40		Windom, 1973
Intertidal sands	<0·010 ⎫ dry		Private communication (DAFS)
Estuarial muds	ca 0·50 ⎭	polluted	
Shoreline sediments:			
Cumberland	0·33–0·60 (dry)	harbour mud	
Morecambe Bay	0·02–0·46 ⎫ dry mean 0·11 ⎬	sand	Private communication (MAFF)
Lancashire Coast	0·02 ⎫ dry 0·25–3·0 ⎬	sand mud	
North Wales Coast	0·3–1·8 (dry)	mud	
Sewage sludges			
UK	1·0–10 ⎫ 2·0–150 ⎬ dry 25–34 ⎭	Glasgow London Manchester	Wood, 1973
UK	150 (dry)		Gardner and Riley, 1973a
Wisconsin	25 (dry)		Syers et al, 1973
Canada	1·0–24 (dry)		van Loon et al, 1973
Sweden	12 (dry)		Andersson and Nilsson, 1972

82

3. Marine sediments

Location and type	Concentration, ppm	Remarks	Reference
Off Cumberland	0·07-0·12 ⎫ dry	mud/sand	Private communication (MAFF)
Morecambe Bay	<0·01-0·04 ⎬	sand	
	0·08-0·29 ⎭	mud	
North Atlantic	0·41 (mean) (dry)		Aston et al, 1972
Torbay	0·02-0·33, mean 0·07 (dry)		Taylor, 1973
Off West Mexico	0·022-0·173	60 km from shore	Weiss et al, 1972
	0·012-0·027	150 km from shore	
Waddenzee	0·25-2·5 (wet)		van Genderen, 1973
New Haven Harbour (Connecticut)	0-2·57 (dry)		Applequist et al, 1972
Santa Barbara Basin	0·04	1500 BP ⎫	Young et al, 1973
	0·060	19th century ⎬ dry	
	0·140	present ⎭	
La Jolla, California	<0·1-1·0		Klein and Goldberg, 1970
Belgian and Danish shoreline	0·1-2, mean 0·3		quoted in Bouquiaux, 1973
Mobile Bay, Alabama	0·21-0·60		Andren and Harriss, 1973
Swedish coastal	1·0-2·0		Ackefors et al, 1970
Minamata Bay, Japan	7·16-801		Saito, 1967
Minamata Bay, Japan	up to 2010 (wet)		Takeuchi, 1972b
	0·4-3·4 outside Bay		

83

REFERENCES

Abbott, D. C. and Tatton, J. O'G., 1970, *Pest. Sci.*, **1**, 99.

Aberg, B., Ekman, L., Falk, R., Greitz, U., Persson, G. and Snihs, J. O., 1969, *Arch. Envir. Hlth.*, **19**, 478.

Ackefors, H., Lofroth, G. and Rosen, G. G., 1970, *Oceanog. Mar. Bio. Ann. Rev.*, **8**, 203.

Akagi, H. and Takabatake, E., 1973, *Chemosphere*, **3**, 131.

Al-Shahristani, H. and Al-Hadaad, I. K., 1973, *J. Radioanal. Chem.*, **15**, 59.

Amin-Zaki, L., Elhassani, S., Majeed, M. A., Clarkson, T. W., Doherty, R. A. and Greenwood, M. R., 1974, 1st International Mercury Congress, Barcelona.

Andersson, A., 1967, *Grundforbattring*, **20**, 95.

Andersson, A. and Nilsson, K. O., 1972, *Ambio*, **1**, 176.

Andren, A. W. and Harriss, R. C., 1973, *Nature* (London), **245**, 256.

Anon, 1973, *Japan Environment Summary*, **1**, 5.

Applequist, M. D., Katz, A. and Turekian, K. K., 1972, *Env. Sci. and Tech.*, **6**, 1123.

Aston, S. R., Bruty, D., Chester, R. and Padgham, R. C., 1973, *Nature* (London), **241**, 450.

Aston, S. R., Bruty, D., Chester, R. and Riley, J. P., 1972, *Nature Physical Science*, **237**, 125.

Auerbach, S. I., 1973, Oak Ridge National Laboratory Environmental Science Division Annual Progress Report, p. 58.

Bache, C. A., et al, 1973, *J. Agr. Fd. Chem.*, **21**, 607.

Bakir, F., Damluji, S. F., Amin-Zaki, L., Murtadha, M., Khalidi, A., Al-Rawi, N. Y., Tikriti, S., Dhahir, H. I., Clarkson, T. W., Smith, J. C. and Doherty, R. A., 1973, *Science*, **181**, 230.

Barber, R. T., Vijayakumar, A. and Cross, F., 1972, *Science*, **178**, 636.

Barr, R. D., Woodger, B. A. and Rees, P. H., 1973, *Am. J. Clin. Path.*, **59**, 36.

Barr, R. D., Smith, H. and Cameron, H. M., 1973b, *Am. J. Clin. Path.*, **59**, 515.

Beck, W. F., et al, 1974, *Nature* (London), **249**, 674.

Ben-Bassatt, D., et al, 1972, *Nature* (London), **240**, 43.

Berg, W., Johnels, A., Sjostrand, B. and Westermark, T., 1966, *Oikos*, **17**, 71.

Berglund, F., et al, 1971, *Nord. Hygien. Tidskr. Suppl.* 4.

Bidstrup, P. L., et al, 1951, *Lancet*, **2**, 856.

Billings, C. E. and Matson, W. R., 1972, *Science,* **176,** 1232.

Bloxam, T. W., Aurora, S. N., Leach, L. and Reas, T. R., 1972, *Nature Physical Science,* **239,** 158.

Bogen, J., 1973, *Atmos. Envt.,* **7,** 1117.

Bombace, M. A., Cigna Rossi, L., Clemente, G. F., Zuccaro Labellarte, G., Allegrini, M. and Lanzola, E., 1973, in 'Problems of the Contamination of Man and His Environment by Mercury and Cadmium'. CEC European Colloquium, Luxembourg, 3–5 July, p. 47.

Borg, K., Wanntorp, H., Erne, K. and Hanko, E., 1969, *Viltrevy,* **6,** 301.

Bouquiaux, J., 1973, in 'Problems of the Contamination of Man and His Environment by Mercury and Cadmium'. CEC European Colloquium, Luxembourg, 3–5 July, p. 23.

Braman, R. S. and Johnson, D. L., 1974, *Env. Sci. and Tech.,* **8,** 996.

Brar, S. S., Nelson, D. M., Kanabroecki, E. L., Moore, C. E., Burnham, C. D. and Hattori, D. M., 1969, NBS Special Publication 312, **1,** 43.

Brobst, D. D. A. and Pratt, W. P., 1973, United States Min. Res. Geol. Sur. Professional Paper 820, 401.

Buckell, M., Hunter, D., Milton, R. and Perry, K. M. A., 1946, *Brit. J. Indust. Med.,* **3,** 55.

Burton, J. D. and Leatherland, T. M., 1971, *Nature,* **231,** 440.

Byrne, A. R., Ravnik, V. and Kosta, L., 1976, *Sci. Tot. Env.,* **6,** 65.

Cadle, R. D., Wartburg, A. F., Pollock, W. H., Gandrud, B. W. and Shedlowsky, J. P., 1973, *Chemosphere,* **6,** 31.

Carr, R. A. and Wilkniss, P. E., 1973, *Science,* **181,** 843.

Carr, R. A., Jones, M. M. and Russ, E. R., 1974, *Nature* (London), **251,** 489.

Childs, A. A., 1973, *Arch. Envir. Hlth.,* **27,** 50.

Cholak, J., 1952, Proc. 2nd Nat. Air Poll. Symp., Pasadena, California.

Clarkson, T. W., 1972, *Ann. Ref. Pharmacol.,* **12,** 375.

Clarkson, T. W., Magos, L. and Greenwood, M. R., 1972, *Biol. Neonate,* **21,** 239.

Clifton, A. P. and Vivian, C. M. G., 1975, *Nature* (London), **253,** 621.

Cook, T. A. and Yates, P. O., 1969, *Brit. Dent. J.,* **127,** 553.

Craig, P. J. and Morton, S. F., 1976, *Nature* (London), **261,** 125.

Curley, A., Sedlak, V. A., Girling, E. F., Hawk, R. E., Barthel, W. F., Pierce, P. E. and Likosky, W. H., 1971, *Science,* **172,** 65.

Cuzacq, G., Comproni, E. M. and Smith, H. L., 1971, *J. Massachusetts Dent. Soc.,* p. 254.

Dale, I. M., Baxter, M. S., Bogan, J. A. and Bourne, W. R. P., 1973, *Mar. Poll. Bull.,* **4,** 77.

Dall'Aglio, M., 1968, in 'Origin and Distribution of the Elements'. *Intern. Earth Sci. Ser, Mon,* **30,** 1065.

Dams, R., Robbins, J. A., Rahn, K. A. and Winchester, J. W., 1970, *Anal. Chem.*, **42**, 861.

Daykin, J. M., 1975, *Vet. Record*, **96**, 255.

Diehl, R. C., et al, 1972, US Bureau of Mines Tech. Prog. Rept. 54.

Dinman, B. D. and Hecker, L. H., 1972, in 'Environmental Mercury Contamination'. Ann Arbor Science Publishers Inc., Ann Arbor, Michigan, p. 291.

Emmelin, L., 1974, *Current Sweden*, No. 49.

Environment Agency, 1975, 'Quality of the Environment in Japan'.

Eriksson, E., 1967, *Oikos*, **9**, 13.

Eshleman, A., Siegel, S. M. and Siegel, B. Z., 1971, *Nature* (London), **233**, 471.

Evans, R. J., Bails, J. D. and d'Itri, F. M., 1972, *Env. Sci. and Tech.*, **6**, 901.

Fimreite, N., Fyfe, R. W. and Keith, J. A., 1970, *Can. Fld. Nat.*, **84**, 269.

Fitzgerald, W. F. and Lyons, W. B., 1973, *Nature* (London), **242**, 452.

Fleischer, M., 1970, in 'Mercury in the Environment'. United States Department of the Interior Geological Survey Professional Paper 713, p. 6.

Foote, R. S., 1972, *Science*, **177**, 513.

Frank, R., et al, 1974, *Can. J. Plant. Sci.*, **54**, 529.

Frear, D. E. H. and Dills, L. E., 1967, *J. Econ. Ent.*, **60**, 970.

Friberg, L., 1951, *Nord. Hyg. Tidskrift*, **32**, 240.

Frissell, M. J., Poelstra, P. and van der Klug, N., 1973, Preprint Paper No. 2 for CEC Colloquium on 'Problems of the Contamination of Man and His Environment by Mercury and Cadmium'. Luxembourg, 3–5 July.

Furukawa, K., et al, 1969, *Agric. Biol. Chem.*, **33**, 128.

Gardner, D., 1975, *Mar. Poll. Bull.*, **6**, 43.

Gardner, D. and Riley, J. P., 1973a, *Est. and Coast. Mar. Sci.*, **1**, 191.

Gardner, D. and Riley, J. P., 1973b, *Nature* (London), **241**, 526.

Gavis, J. and Ferguson, J. F., 1972, *Wat. Res.*, **6**, 989.

van Genderen, H., 1973, in 'Problems of the Contamination of Man and His Environment by Mercury and Cadmium'. CEC Colloquium, Luxembourg, 3–5 July, p. 247.

Gibbs, R. H., Jarosewich, E. and Windom, H. L., 1974, *Science*, **184**, 475.

de Goeij, J. J. and Houtman, J. P. W., 1971, *Chem. Weekblad*, **67**, 13.

Goldberg, E. D., 1968, in 'Global Effects of Environmental Pollution', D. Reidel Publishing Company, Dordrecht-Holland, p. 178.

Goldberg, E. D. and Gross, M. G., 1971, in 'Man's Impact on Terrestrial and Oceanic Ecosystems'. MIT Press, Cambridge, Massachusetts, p. 371.

Goldwater, L. J., 1965, *J. Fd. Cosmet. Toxicol*, **3**, 120.

Goldwater, L. J., 1971, *Scientific American,* **224,** 15.

Goldwater, L. J. and Clarkson, T. W., 1972, in 'Metallic Contaminants and Human Health', Academic Press, New York, p. 17.

Gracey, H. I. and Stewart, J. W. B., 1974, *Can. J. Soil. Sci.,* **54,** 105.

Greenwood, M. R., Clarkson, T. W. and Magos, L., 1972, *Experientia,* **28,** 1455.

Gronka, P. A., Bobkoskie, R. L., Tomchick, G. J., Bach, F. and Rakow, A. B., 1970, *J. Am. Dent. Ass.,* **81,** 923.

Hammerston, R. J., Hissong, D. E., Kopfler, F. C., Mayer, J., McFarren, E. F. and Pringle, B. H., 1972, *J. Am. Wat. Wks. Ass.,* p. 60.

Harris, L. H., 1972, Ph.D. Thesis, Michigan University, 'Hair as an Index of Mercury and Lead Exposure'.

Hasanen, E., 1973, in 'Problems of the Contamination of Man and His Environment by Mercury and Cadmium'. CEC Colloquium, 3–5 July, Luxembourg, p. 109.

Hasselrot, T. B., 1968, Report of the Institute of Freshwater Research, Drottningholm, **48,** 102.

Hecker, L. H., Allen, H. E., Dinman, B. D. and Neel, J. V., 1974, *Arch. Envir. Hlth.,* **29,** 181.

Heide, F., Lerz, H. and Bohm, G., 1957, *Naturwissenschafte,* **44,** 441.

Heindryckx, R., Demuynck, M., Dams, R., Janssens, M. and Ralm, K. A., 1973, in 'Problems of the Contamination of Man and His Environment by Mercury and Cadmium'. CEC Colloquium, Luxembourg, 3–5 July, p. 135.

Heppelstone, P. B. and French, M. C., 1973, *Nature* (London), **243,** 302.

Hewett, P. D., 1974, ADAS Quarterly Review.

HMSO, 1970, 'Taken for Granted'. Report of the Working Party on Sewage Disposal.

HMSO, 1971, Survey of Mercury in Food.

HMSO, 1972, 109th Annual Report on Alkali, &c Works.

HMSO, 1973, 'Out of Sight, Out of Mind'. Report of a Working Party on the Disposal of Sludge in Liverpool Bay, Volume 3.

HMSO, 1973a, Survey of Mercury in Food: A Supplementary Report.

HMSO, 1973b, Threshold Limit Values for 1973. Technical Data Note 2/73, Department of Employment, HM Factory Inspectorate.

HMSO, 1974a, 'The Monitoring of the Environment in the United Kingdom'. Pollution Paper No. 1, Department of the Environment, Central Unit on Environmental Pollution.

HMSO, 1974b, 'The Non-agricultural Uses of Pesticides in Great Britain'. Pollution Paper No. 3, Department of the Environment, Central Unit on Environmental Pollution.

Holden, A. V., 1972, in 'Mercury Contamination in Man and His Environment', International Atomic Energy Agency, Vienna. Technical Report Series No. 137, p. 143.

Holden, A. V., 1973, *J. Fd. Tech.* **8,** 1.

Holden, A. V. and Topping, G., 1972, *Proc. Roy. Soc. Edin.,* **71,** 189.

Holdgate, M. W. (ed), 1971, 'The Seabird Wreck of 1969 in the Irish Sea', Natural Environment Research Council, London.

Hosohara, K., 1961, *Nippon Kagaku Zasshi*, **82**, 1107.

Hosohara, K., Kuroda, R. and Hamaguchi, H., 1961, *Nippon Kagaku Zasshi*, **82**, 347.

Howie, R. A. and Smith, H., 1967, *J. Forensic Sci. Soc.*, **7**, 90.

Japan Times, 1973, 24 May.

Jefferies, D. J. and French, M. C., 1976, *Env. Poll.*, **10**, 175.

Jenne, E. A., 1970, in 'Mercury in the Environment', United States Department of the Interior Geological Survey Professional Paper 713, p. 40.

Jensen, S. and Jernelov, A., 1972, in 'Mercury Contamination in Man and His Environment', International Atomic Energy Agency, Vienna. Technical Report Series No. 137, p. 43.

Jernelov, A., 1972, in 'The Changing Chemistry of the Oceans', Wiley Interscience Division, John Wiley and Sons Inc., New York, London and Sydney, p. 161.

Jernelov, A. and Wallin, T., 1973, *Atmos. Env.*, **7**, 209.

Joensuu, O. I., 1971, *Science*, **172**, 1027.

Johnels, A. G., Westermark, T., Berg, W., Persson, P. I. and Sjöstrand, B., 1967, *Oikos*, **18**, 323.

Johnson, D. L. and Braman, R. S., 1974, *Env. Sci. and Tech.*, **8**, 1003.

Jonasson, I. R., 1973, *Nature* (London), **241**, 447.

Jones, H. R., 1971, in 'Mercury Pollution Control', Noyes Data Corporation, p. 165.

Jones, P., 1975, 'Trace Metals and other Elements in Crude Oil: a Literature Review', British Petroleum Co. Ltd.

Jones, P. and Nickless, G., 1973, *Proc. Soc. Anal. Chem.*, **10**, 269.

Kamps, L. R., Carr, R. and Miller, H., 1972, *Bull. Env. Contam. Tox.*, **8**, 273.

Kempf, T., 1973, in 'Problems of the Contamination of Man and His Environment by Mercury and Cadmium'. CEC Colloquium, Luxembourg, 3–5 July, p. 121.

Kennedy, E. J., Ruch, R. R., Gluskoter, H. J. and Shrimp, N. F., 1971, in Proc. Symposium on Nuclear Methods in Environmental Research, University of Missouri, Columbia, p. 205.

Kibukamusoke, J. W., Davies, D. R. and Hull, M. S. R., 1974, *Br. Med. J.*, No. 5920, 646.

Kim, L.-Y., et al, 1970, *Fac. Pharm. Sci. Univ. Tokyo.*

Kimura, Y. and Miller, V. L., 1964, *J. Agr. Fd. Chem.*, **12**, 253.

Klein, D. H., 1972, *J. Chem. Educ.*, **49**, 7.

Klein, D. H. and Goldberg, E. D., 1970, *Env. Sci. and Tech.*, **4**, 765.

Klein, D. H. and Russell, P. 1973, *Env. Sci. and Tech.*, **7**, 357.

Kloke, A. and Schenke, H. D., 1973, in 'Problems of the Contamination of Man and His Environment by Mercury and Cadmium'. CEC Colloquium, Luxembourg, 3–5 July, p. 83.

Knight, L. A. and Herring, J., 1972, *Pest Monit. J.* (Atlanta), **6**, 103.

Koeman, J. H., Peeters, W., Kondstall-Hol, C., Tjioe, P. and de Goeij, J., 1973, *Nature* (London), **245**, 285.

Kosta, L., Byrne, A. R. and Zelenko, V., 1975, *Nature* (London), **254**, 238.

Krenkel, P. A., 1974, *Crit. Rev. Env. Cont.*, **4**, 251.

Kudsk, F. N., 1965, *Acta. Pharmacol. Toxicol*, **23**, 250.

Kudsk, F. N., 1969, *Acta. Pharmacol. Toxicol.*, **27**, 149.

Leatherland, T. M., Burton, J. D., McCartney, M. J. and Culkin, F., 1971, *Nature* (London), **232**, 112.

Lenihan, J. M. A., Smith, H. and Harvey, W., 1973, *Br. Dent. J.*, **135**, 365.

Lockeretz, W., 1974, *Water, Air and Soil Poll.*, **3**, 179.

van Loon, J. C., 1974, *Env. Letts.*, **6**, 211.

van Loon, J. C., Lichwa, J., Ruttan, D. and Kinrade, J., 1973, *Water, Air and Soil Poll.*, **2**, 473.

Lord, K. A., et al, 1971, *Pest. Sci.*, **2**, 49.

Mackay, N. J., Kazacos, M. N., Williams, R. J. and Leedow, M. I., 1975, *Mar. Poll. Bull.*, **6**, 57.

MacLean, A. J., et al, 1973, *Can. J. Soil Sci.*, **53**, 130.

Magos, L., 1968, *Br. J. Indust. Med.*, **25**, 325.

Martin, J. T., 1963, *Analyst*, **88**, 413.

Mastromatteo, E. and Sutherland, R. B., 1972, in 'Environmental Mercury Contamination', Ann Arbor Science Publishers, Ann Arbor, Michigan, p. 86.

Mayz, E., Corn, M. and Barry, G., 1971, *Am. Ind. Hyg. Ass. J.*, **32**, 373.

McCarthy, J. H., Meuschke, J. L., Ficklin, W. H. and Learned, R. E., 1970, in 'Mercury in the Environment', United States Department of the Interior Geological Survey Professional Paper 713, p. 37.

Miettinen, J. K., et al, 1971, *Ann. Clin. Res.*, **3**, 116

Miller, S. L., Domey, R. G., Elston, S. F. and Milligan, G., 1974, *J. Am. Dent. Ass.*, **89**, 1084.

Miller, G. E., Grant, P. M., Kishore, R., Steinkruger, F. J., Rowland, F. S. and Gunn, V. P., 1972, *Science*, **175**, 1121.

Monier-Williams, G. W., 1949, 'Trace Elements in Food', Chapman and Hall, London.

Mottet, N. K. and Body, R. L., 1974, *Arch. Envir. Hlth.*, **29**, 18.

Neville, G. A., 1967, *Can. Chem. Education*, **3**, 4.

Nuzzi, R., 1972, *Nature* (London), **237**, 38.

Ohta, Y., 1966, *Japan J. Ind. Hlth.*, **8**, 12.

Olafsson, J., 1975, *Nature* (London), **255**, 138.

Olsson, M., 1976, *Ambio*, **5**, 73.

Parslow, J. L. F., 1973a, *Lundy Fld. Soc. Ann. Rept.*, **23**, 31.

Parslow, J. L. F., 1973b, *Env. Poll.*, **5**, 295.

Parslow, J. L. F., Jefferies, D. J. and French, M. C., 1972, *Bird Study*, **19**, 18.

Parslow, J. L. F., Jefferies, D. J. and Hanson, H. M., 1973, *Mar. Poll. Bull.*, **4**, 41.

Peakall, D. B. and Lovett, R. J., 1972, *Bioscience*, **22**, 20.

Peirson, D. H., Cawse, P. A., Salmon, L. and Cambray, R. S., 1973, *Nature* (London), **241**, 252.

Pillay, K. K. S., Thomas, C. G., Sondel, J. A. and Hyche, C. M., 1972, *Env. Res.*, **5**, 172.

Poelstra, P., et al, 1973, *Neth. J. Agr. Sci.*, **21**, 77.

Portmann, J. E., 1974, in United States Environmental Protection Agency/State University of New Jersey Symposium on 'Pretreatment and Ultimate Disposal of Wastewater Solids', State University of New Jersey, 21–22 May.

Portmann, J. E. and Wilson, K. W., 1971, Ministry of Agriculture, Fisheries and Food Laboratory Leaflet No. 22.

Raeder, M. G. and Snekvik, E., 1940, *K. Vidensk Selsk, Forh.*, **13**, 169.

Rancitelli, L. A., 1971, Pacific Northwest Laboratory Annual Report to USAEC Division of Biology and Medicine. Vol. II. Physical Sciences, Pt. 2. Radiological Sciences, Battelle Memorial Institute, Richland, Washington, Environmental and Life Sciences Division, p. 37.

Recht, P., Smeets, J., Amavis, R. and Berlin, A., in 'Problems of the Contamination of Man and His Environment by Mercury and Cadmium'. CEC Colloquium, Luxembourg, 3–5 July, p. 673.

Rivers, J. B., Pearson, J. E. and Shultz, C. D., 1972, *Bull. Env. Contam. Tox.*, **8**, 257.

Rook, H. L., LaFleur, P. D. and Gills, T. E., 1972, *Env. Lett.*, **2**, 195.

Rossi, L. C., Clemente, G. F. and Santaroni, G., 1976, *Arch. Env. Hlth.*, **31**, 160.

Ruch, R. R., Gluskoter, H. J. and Kennedy, E. J., 1971, *Env. Geol. Notes*, No. 43, 1.

Saha, J. G., et al, 1970, *Can. J. Plant Sci.*, **50**, 597.

Saito, N., 1967, Intern. At. Energy Authority Symposium, Amsterdam.

Sartor, J. D., Boyd, G. B. and Agardy, F. J., 1974, *J. Wat. Poll. Con. Fed.*, **46**, 458.

Schlesinger, M. D. and Schultz, H., 1971, US Bureau of Mines, Technical Program Report 43.

Schramel, P., Samsahl, K. and Pavlu, J., 1973, *Int. J. Env. Studies*, **5**, 37.

Selikoff, I. J., 1971, *Env. Res.*, **4**, 1.

Shacklette, H. T., et al, 1971, US Geol. Survey. Circular No. 644.

Siegel, B. Z., Siegel, S. M. and Thorarinsson, F., 1973, *Nature* (London), **241**, 526.

Siegel, S. M., Siegel, B. Z., Eshlemann, A. M. and Bachman, K., 1973b, *Env. Biol. and Med.*, **2**, 81.

Sikes, C. S. and Drain, M. P., 1973, *Nature*, **224**, 529.

Simpson, R. E., Horwitz, W. and Roy, C. A., 1974, *Pest. Monit. J.*, **7**, 127.

Skerfving, S., Hansson, K. and Lindsten, J., 1970, *Arch. Envir. Hlth.*, **21**, 133.

Smith, J. D., Nicholson, R. A. and Moore, P. J., 1971, *Nature* (London), **232**, 393.

Smith, W. E. and Smith, A. M., 1975, 'Minamata', Chatto and Windus, London.

Spangler, W. J., Spigarelli, J. L., Rose, J. M. and Miller, H. M., 1973, *Science*, **180**, 192.

Stanley, P. I. and Elliott, G. R., 1976, *Agro-Ecosystems*, **2**, 223.

Stegner, P., Kosta, L., Byrne, A. R. and Ravnik, V., 1973, *Chemosphere*, **2**, 57.

Stein, P. C., Campbell, E. E., Moss, W. D. and Trujillo, P., 1974, *Arch. Envir. Hlth.*, **29**, 25.

Stijve, T. and Roschnik, R., 1974, *Trav. Chim. Aliment. Hyg.*, **65**, 209.

Stock, A. and Cucuel, F., 1934a, *Naturwissenschaften*, **22**, 390.

Stock, A. and Cucuel, F., 1934b, *Deut. Chem. Ges., Ber.*, **67B**, 122.

Strickland, A. H., 1967, Proc. 4th Brit. Ins. and Fung. Conf., **2**, 478.

Sumari, P., Partanen, T., Heitala, S. and Heinonen, O. P., 1972, *Work-environment Health*, **9**, 61.

Sumner, A. K., Saha, J. G. and Lee, Y. W., 1972, *Pest. Monit. J.*, **6**, 122.

Suzuki, T., Matsumoto, N., Miyama, T. and Katsunuma, H., 1967, *Ind. Hlth.* (Japan), **5**, 149.

Syers, J. K., Iskandor, I. K. and Keeney, D. R., 1973, *Water, Air and Soil Poll.*, **2**, 105.

Takeuchi, T., 1972a, in 'Environmental Mercury Contamination', Ann Arbor Science Publishers Inc., Ann Arbor, Michigan, p. 247.

Takeuchi, T., 1972b, Ibid, p. 79.

Takeuchi, T., 1972c, Ibid, p. 302.

Tanner, T. M., Young, T. A. and Cooper, J. A., 1974, *Chemosphere*, **3**, 211.

Taylor, C. J., to be published.

Taylor, D., 1973, ICI Brixham Laboratory Report BL/B/1448.

Tejning, S., 1967, *Oikos.*, Suppl. 8, 1–116.

Tonomura, K., Maeda, K. and Futai, F., 1968, *J. Ferment. Technol.*, **46**, 506.

Topping, G. and Pirie, J. M., 1972, *Anal. Chem. Acta.*, **62**, 200.

Turner, M. D., Marsh, D. O., Rubio, C. E., Chiriboga, J., Chiriboga, C. C., Smith J. C. and Clarkson, T. W., 1974, 1st International Mercury Congress, Barcelona.

Warren, H. V. and Delavault, R. E., 1969, *Oikos*, **20**, 537.

Weiss, H. V., Koide, M. and Goldberg, E. D., 1971, *Science*, **174**, 692.

Weiss, H. V., Yamamoto, S., Crozier, T. E. and Matthewson, J. H., 1972, *Env. Sci. and Tech.*, **6**, 644.

Welsh Office, 1975, Report of a Collaborative Study on Certain Elements in Air, Soil, Plants, Animals and Humans in the Swansea-Neath-Port Talbot area, together with a Report on a Moss-Bag Study of Atmospheric Pollution across South Wales.

Wershaw, R. L., 1970, in 'Mercury in the Environment', United States Department of the Interior Geological Survey Professional Paper 713, p. 29.

Westermark, T., Odsjo, T. and Johnels, A. G., 1975, *Ambio*, **4**, 87.

White, D. E., Hinkle, M. E. and Barnes, I., 1970, in 'Mercury in the Environment', United States Department of the Interior Geological Survey Professional Paper 713, p. 25.

Wilcox, K. R., 1972, in 'Environmental Mercury Contamination', Ann Arbor Science Publishers Inc., Ann Arbor, Michigan, p. 82.

Williston, S. H., 1968, *J. Geophys. Res.*, **73**, 7051.

Windom, H. L., 1973, *Journal of the Waterways, Harbours and Coastal Engineering Division*, **99**, 257.

WHO, 1972, Health Hazards of the Human Environment, 185. Geneva, 1972.

WHO, 1972a, World Health Organisation Food Additive Series, No. 4, Geneva, 1972.

WHO, 1974, World Health Organisation Technical Report Series No. 555, Geneva, 1974.

Wood, P. C., 1973, in 'Proceedings of National Symposium on Disposal of Municipal and Industrial Sludges and Solid Trade Wastes', London, 26–27 November, Paper No. 8.

Wroblewski, S. C., Spittler, T. M. and Harrison, P. R., 1974, *J. Air Poll. Cont. Ass.*, **24**, 778.

Yamada, M. and Tonomura, K., 1972, *J. Ferment. Technol.*, **50**, 159.

Young, D. R., Johnson, J. N., Soutar, A. and Isaacs, J. D., 1973, *Nature* (London), **244**, 273.

Zimmerman, P. W. and Crocker, W., 1933, Boyce Thomson Inst. Professional Papers, **1**, No. 23, 222.

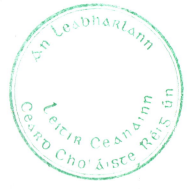

Printed in England for Her Majesty's Stationery Office by The White Rose Press, Mexborough and London
Dd. 587454 9/76 K36